SH03004682
23-7-04

WITHDRAWN

D0302584

Fundamental Aspects of
Palliative Care Nursing

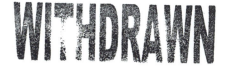

WITHDRAWN

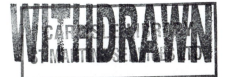

WITHDRAWN
CARDIFF
STAFF LIBRARY

Other titles published by Quay Books, MA Healthcare Limited, in the 'Fundamental Aspects of Nursing' series:

Fundamental Aspects of Legal, Ethical and Professional Issues in Nursing by Maggie Reeves and Jacquie Orford
Fundamental Aspects of Women's Health by Morag Gray
Fundamental Aspects of Men's Health by Morag Gray
Fundamental Aspects of Tissue Viability by Cheryl Dunford and Bridget Günnewicht

series editor: John Fowler

Fundamental Aspects of Palliative Care Nursing

Robert Becker and Richard Gamlin

Quay Books
MA Healthcare Limited

Quay Books Division, MA Healthcare Limited, Jesses Farm, Snow Hill, Dinton, Salisbury, Wiltshire, SP3 5HN

British Library Cataloguing-in-Publication Data
A catalogue record is available for this book

© MA Healthcare Limited 2004
ISBN 1 85642 211 9

All rights reserved. No part of this publication may be reproduced, stored in a retrieval system or transmitted in any form or by any means, electronic, mechanical, photocopying, recording or otherwise, without prior permission from the publishers

Printed in the UK by Cromwell Press, Trowbridge

Contents

Preface

The first time that Bob and I taught together in Russia, I watched him as he explained the philosophy of palliative care. 'Palliative care is a blend of the head, the hands and the heart', said Bob pointing in turn to his head, his hands and his heart. 'The most important of these is the heart', he continued. This was one of the most powerful teaching moments I have ever witnessed. Our students immediately understood the significance of his words and gestures. I have used this approach many times since, in this country and abroad, to stimulate a philosophical debate about the art and science of palliative care.

This is the essence of palliative care, and the more I think about it, the essence of life. In this book we have attempted to achieve a balance between the head, the hands and the heart. If you go with your heart, you will rarely go wrong.

I have been passionate about palliative care for about thirty-five years. It has taught me so much more about life than it has about death. In *Chapter 8* we discuss handling difficult questions. Perhaps the question, 'How long have I got?' is the most challenging of them all. When I have explored this question with patients they usually tell me that, in the time that is left, they wish to accomplish something which has always been important to them but, for one reason or another, they have just not got round to it. If you think like this please don't wait until you are dying to reach for those goals. Do it now!

Richard Gamlin

There are no easy answers to the complex dilemmas in end of life care that we meet in our increasingly medicalised healthcare environment. As nurses we seem to spend more and more of our time searching for definitive factual evidence that the package of palliative care we offer our patients and their family actually works, when the real answers are there on the faces and in the words and actions of the people who have been helped.

If, as you read this book and use it in clinical practice, it helps you bring the combination of head, hands and heart together then you will know that you have truly made a difference to someone's life. You will also begin to appreciate that it is not always quantifiable by using assessment tools, grading points and statistics.

I know that some of the most inspirational palliative care that I have witnessed has been in destitute and poverty stricken environments, where the science that western medicine takes for granted has mostly been unavailable. These nurses have had no option but to use whatever is at hand and their natural intuitive abilities. I can assure you that they most certainly make a difference to people's lives. Learning the lessons from such encounters is at the heart of good nursing so, to paraphrase the words of Derek Doyle (1999), we should stop filling the heads of our students with facts and figures, doses and data, and instead concentrate on trying to shape attitudes by sharing with our students some of the profound insights into the human condition which so characterise palliative care.

Robert Becker

Reference

Doyle D (1999) Upon Reflection: A farewell address. *Supportive Care in Cancer* **8**(2): 77–9

Foreword

As a student nurse at the end of my training and about to embark on my nursing career, I enjoyed reading *Fundamental Aspects of Palliative Care Nursing*, and feel honoured to have been asked to write a foreword. It was a highly readable text, interesting with case studies throughout, and can be used as a handy reference guide with its practical bullet points. The book defines palliative care, and addresses some of the more difficult aspects of this area of nursing, for example: ethical issues surrounding the care of the terminally ill; caring for the bereaved before and after the death of their loved ones, and communicating with patients who are facing death. It even offers suggestions for what to say in these difficult situations. In addition, the authors explore spiritual care, which is not an easy concept for newly qualified nurses.

On a practical level, it offers evidence-based research and suggestions for achieving quality care for the terminally ill. What particularly impressed me while reading the book were the practical suggestions for the assessment and relief of pain and other distressing symptoms of advanced illness, and how to provide the best possible basic patient care. The latter made me realise that this is how nurses should care for all patients, in all settings.

The book has been written by experts who have knowledge, experience, and a passionate interest in the field of palliative care, and reflected back to me what I had seen and experienced during one of my student placements at a hospice. A useful text not only for students and nurses with an interest in palliative care, but for those in any area of nursing, as distress, serious illness, and death, do not confine themselves to the palliative care setting.

Debra Fear
Student Nurse
Staffordshire University School of Health

When I was approached to write the foreword for *Fundamental Aspects of Palliative Care Nursing* I felt very honoured. As I am on the brink of qualifying as an adult nurse and embarking on my nursing career, reading the text enabled me to reflect and re-evaluate a number of incidents which occurred while in the hospital environment.

For example, I once encountered a courageous young woman who was trying to come to terms with her terminal diagnosis. Her family were very distraught; in particular, her mother who approached me and asked if it was wrong of her to want her daughter's suffering to end. I am aware that families/friends to an extent do grieve before the anticipated death of a loved one. I sat with the mother as she talked and we cried about the impending loss of her only child. *Chapter 7,* 'Caring for the bereaved' stood out in my mind, as it helped me to reflect on this particular incident and to confirm that what I did was good practice.

I found the case studies within the text inspiring, and they acted as a catalyst for me to reflect on my work with the dying so far, and to challenge my actions and question my motives.

I have read various palliative care books but this one is different and I personally believe that it is directed at the correct level for junior members of staff and offers information, which is patient-centred, relevant and informative from a nursing perspective.

Chapter 5, 'Managing symptoms other than pain' made me aware that patients' pain may not just be from a physical origin. There may be other underlying factors, such as the patient's position, mattress or psychological, spiritual and social factors, which cause pain. I was impressed to see at the end of each chapter the referenced links to the Nursing and Midwifery Council's (NMC's) *Code of Professional Conduct* and various other topic areas used within the chapters. These references enable you to stimulate your self-awareness and facilitate learning, particularly for student nurses and healthcare assistants.

Overall, I consider *Fundamental Aspects of Palliative Care Nursing* to be an excellent text, which is oriented towards all junior members of the multidisciplinary team, not just within palliative care but within all aspects of nursing/patient care.

Tracy Fisher
Student Nurse
Staffordshire University School of Health

Introduction

Caring for those who are dying and their families has long been recognised as an immensely challenging and stressful part of health and social care (Vachon, 1988; Benner and Wrubel, 1989). Doing it well in today's complex, increasingly secular, and politically oriented healthcare culture poses as many challenges for nurses now as it did in the pioneering days of the palliative care movement in the early 1960s. Those challenges are significantly different to the ones faced some forty years ago. The science of palliative care has developed rapidly and continues to do so, due mostly to the central role of pharmacological interventions to help control chronic pain and distressing symptoms. This is a vital and essential aspect of optimising the patient's quality of life, and has undoubtedly contributed to the wide acceptance of palliative care as a recognised medical speciality world-wide.

The art of caring, however, has received significantly less attention over the years, perhaps because of its more abstract nature. It is much more difficult to provide demonstrable clinical evidence of the success of interpersonal interventions to the overall quality of care to someone who is dying when the outcome is death itself.

Underpinning this is the declaration of the World Health Organization defining palliative care which was first published in 1990 and has recently been updated in 2002. This definition remains a landmark statement, as it not only helped to clarify the goals of care, but also emphasised to all professional carers that they need to think and act holistically, towards both patient and family, and view dying as a normal life event, rather than one dominated by the disease process.

Thereby lies the paradox and the challenge to those involved in end of life care. How to marry up the art and the science into a cohesive approach that reflects individuality, choice, dignity, and compassion in whatever environment the care takes place.

The aim of this book is to provide a concise practical resource text to nurses and students of nursing that emphasises the art and science of palliative care in tandem. A book that sees 'caring' as the fundamental underpinning and overarching concept to successful practice in whatever clinical environment they may work. The intention is to move away from the somewhat exaggerated emphasis on the contribution of physicians to patient care within the literature currently available, when in reality the vast majority of care given in this field is the domain of other disciplines, and amongst those nursing is the most numerous (Barnard *et al*, 2000).

Any book that discusses the practice of palliative care needs to acknowledge the contribution of the many other disciplines involved in the patient and family's experience during such a difficult life crisis. Of all the diverse areas of care that exist in our healthcare system, few have grappled with, and achieved as much towards the reality of true interdisciplinary working, as the field of palliative care, a fact that is readily acknowledged world-wide.

The emphasis in this book is on making the reader aware of the extensive material that currently exists that is accepted good practice, rather than providing a detailed meta analysis of theoretical and research-based concepts. There are already a few, excellent texts on the market which attempt to do this from a nursing perspective (Kinghorn and Gamlin, 2001; Lugton and Kindlen, 1999; Aranda and O'Connor, 2003) and both are in many respects essential reading to complement academic studies in the field.

For many nurses, there are often occasions in clinical practice when they ask themselves:

> *What advice, techniques, suggestions, or interventions*
> *can I use at this moment to enhance care?*

The next question often is:

> *What was it that was said in that lecture/course I*
> *attended about this situation? I wish I could*
> *remember and I had the handouts close by...*

It is simply not possible, of course, to go to a locker or the boot of a car at sensitive, difficult moments to look for resources and, indeed, it is inappropriate to do so. It is possible, however, to carry with you one compact text, which offers comprehensive, evidence-based, practice guidelines across the spectrum of palliative care scenarios to provide a trigger and opportunity for reflection and learning. This is where this book fits.

Each chapter examines a key component of care and is supported by appropriate evidence-based references and links to the NMC's *Code of Professional Conduct* (2002). Worldwide web and electronic resources that closely link to the chapter theme are also included.

To have the opportunity to be at the bedside of someone throughout the final moments of their life is indeed a privilege and honour for any carer. To attempt to analyse and define this in quantifiable terms is perhaps rather like looking for the pot of gold at the end of the rainbow. This book makes no false pretensions along that road, but it can become a useful spanner in the toolbox of skills, knowledge and compassion that nurses draw on, in, what is inevitably, an emotive and sensitive life event. Moreover, it can be an aid and boost to confidence, to that most undervalued yet essential quality which helps a nurse understand the value of 'being' as well as 'doing' in our busy clinical environments.

References

Aranda S, O'Connor M (2003) *Palliative Care Nursing: A guide to practice.* Radcliffe Medical Press, Oxford

Barnard D, Towers A, Boston P, Lambrindou Y (2000) *Crossing Over: Narratives of Palliative Care.* Oxford University Press, Oxford

Benner P, Wrubel (1989) *The Primacy of Care.* Addison Wesley, California

Lugton J, Kindlen M (1999) *Palliative Care: The Nursing Role.* Churchill Livingstone, London

Kinghorn S, Gamlin R (2001) *Palliative Nursing: Bringing comfort and hope.* Baillière Tindall, London

Vachon M (1988) Battle fatigue in hospice and palliative care. In: Gilmore A, Gilmore S, eds. *A Safer Death* . Plenum Press, New York

World Health Organization (1990) *Cancer Pain Relief and Palliative Care.* Technical Report Series 804. Report of the WHO expert committee, Geneva

World Health Organization (2002) *National Cancer Control Programmes: Policies and Managerial Guidelines.* 2nd edn. WHO, Geneva,

Useful websites

World Health Organization
http://www.who.int/cancer

National Hospice Council
http://www.hospice-spc-council.org.uk

Acknowledgements

We would like to acknowledge the help, support and encouragement given to us over the last two years while this book has taken shape. In particular, we would like to thank the publishers for their investment of faith in our initial idea, the reviewers who guided us and our loved ones for their support and tolerance when the going got tough. Thanks and dedication must also go to a small group of trusted colleagues and wise friends who have inspired and influenced us over the years, and have helped mould the values and beliefs that underpin our work as teachers of palliative care.

Dedication

For those with whom I have shared love. You have brought meaning to my life and helped to shape me into who I have become. There are no words. I thank you from the bottom of my heart.

Richard Gamlin

Chapter I

What is palliative care nursing?

In order to truly understand the nature of palliative care nursing and exactly what it is attempting to achieve it is necessary to take a brief, but thorough look at what has been said so far about the concepts of palliation, nursing and caring.

Nursing

There have been many definitions of nursing published over the last fifty years but in the context of palliative care, perhaps the most succinct is that written by Virginia Henderson (1997):

> *Nursing is primarily assisting the individual in the performance of those activities contributing to health and its recovery, or to a peaceful death.*

The key phrases that stand out in this definition from a palliative viewpoint are:

> *... assisting the individual... to a peaceful death.*

The inference is one of partnership, helping, and dignity.

Palliative

The word 'palliative' has its origins in the Latin word pallium, meaning a cloak or cover, but a more contemporary and simple definition is, 'to mitigate the sufferings of the patient, not to effect a cure' as offered by the *Blacks Medical Dictionary* (Macpherson, 1992).

The discipline of palliative care has also been defined by numerous organisations, each contributing its own standpoint (World Health Organization [WHO], 1990, 2002; European Association of Palliative Care [EAPC], 1989; National Council for Hospice and Specialist Palliative Care Services [NCHSPCS], 1995, 2001).

Perhaps the most widely known and accepted is that produced by the World Health Organization (2002):

> *Palliative care is an approach that improves the quality of life of patients and their families facing the problem associated with life-threatening illness, through the prevention and relief of suffering by means of early identification and impeccable assessment and treatment of pain and other problems, physical, psychosocial and spiritual.*

⌘ *provides relief from pain and other distressing symptoms*

⌘ *affirms life and regards dying as a normal process*

⌘ *intends neither to hasten nor postpone death; integrates the psychological and spiritual aspects of patient care*

⌘ *offers a support system to help patients live as actively as possible until death*

⌘ *offers a support system to help the family cope during the patient's illness and in their own bereavement*

⌘ *uses a team approach to address the needs of patients and their families, including bereavement counselling, if indicated*

⌘ *will enhance quality of life, and may also positively influence the course of illness*

⌘ *is applicable early in the course of illness, in conjunction with other therapies that are intended to prolong life, such as chemotherapy or radiation therapy, and includes those investigations needed to better understand and manage distressing clinical complications.*

The key phrases and words that stand out from this definition are:

- improves the quality of life of patients and their families
- the prevention and relief of suffering
- relief from pain and other distressing symptoms
- regards dying as a normal process
- neither to hasten or postpone death
- offers a support system... patient and family.

The inference in this definition is similar to Virginia Henderson's (1997), but there is a clear and expanded emphasis on holism, quality of life, normality and support for both patient and family. All these aims are consistent with good nursing practice and can help us to conceptualise what nurses should be attempting to achieve when they have contact with the dying and bereaved.

Care

What then of the concept of 'care'? A number of authors have attempted to discover what this means to those delivering care and those receiving it. Others have attempted to analyse this complex phenomenon and it is worth looking at what has been said, as the act of caring is widely recognised as the underpinning philosophy central to all nursing practice (Morse *et al*, 1991). Nurses do not have a monopoly on caring, nor do they occupy the moral high ground in this area; but nurses are in a unique situation as the only twenty-four-hour carers in the healthcare system to embrace and develop this concept if they choose to do so. We venture to suggest that if a clearer understanding of the basis of caring is integrated into practice, then it is indeed possible to achieve the principles of the palliative approach in multiple environments.

There is ample evidence that a caring approach is effective and is valued by both patients and families. For example:

⌘ Reiman (1986) investigated patients' descriptions of non-caring nurse behaviour. The main factor contributing to this was the physical and emotional distance of the nurse.

⌘ Forest (1989) investigated nurse perceptions of caring. The results indicated that caring is a, 'mental and emotional presence that comes from deep feelings for the patients' experience'.

⌘ Brown (1986) investigated hospital patients' views of caring. The results showed that the most important quality to the patient's experience of care was the reassuring presence of the nurse.

⌘ Hinds, Martin and Vogel (1987) explored hopefulness in young oncology patients. A key finding was that they saw the nurses' personal commitment to a relationship with them as evidence of caring.

The key words that emerge from this research are: closeness, presence, emotional involvement and relationships. These words are closely allied to those expressed by Roach (1987), Mayeroff (2003) and Watson (1985) whose theories used words, such as:

ℋ Patience, honesty, trust, humility, hope, courage, compassion, competence, conscience, commitment, altruism, faith, spirituality, relationships, supportive, sensitivity, problem solving, teaching, and learning.

It is these adjectives and qualities, which perhaps epitomise the real role of a nurse as perceived by those receiving the care.

Palliative nursing can make a difference

ℋ We know that patients tell us that they wish to be more involved in treatment decisions (National Cancer Alliance [NCA], 1996).

ℋ Patients and relatives tell nurses what they value most about the care they receive (Manley, 1988).

ℋ When chemotherapy, radiotherapy and immunotherapy are delivered and completed it is nurses who mostly bear the burden of care (Kearney, 1999).

ℋ There is clear evidence available that good nursing care has a positive effect on quality of life for our patients (Smith and Sttullenbarger, 1995; Corner *et al*, 1999; Macintosh and Bowles, 1997).

Why do nurses find palliative care difficult?

Twenty reasons:

1. We don't have enough staff where I work.
2. I don't have the time to deal with the complex issues involved.
3. there are too many other important priorities in my job.
4. I don't have the skills to deal with it.
5. I don't have the knowledge of drugs and symptom control.
6. I don't know what to say to patients and relatives when they ask difficult questions.
7. I'm afraid they might get upset.
8. I'm afraid I might get upset.
9. Getting upset means I can't do my job properly.
10. I haven't done a course on the subject yet.
11. I just find the whole business too much to deal with.
12. I'm afraid that I might get into trouble with senior staff if I spend too much time around the bedside and I haven't got a task to perform.

13. If something goes wrong, I'm afraid I might get the blame.
14. I've never had a major loss myself so how can I ever expect to understand and help someone who is dying.
15. This is just not the right place for someone to die, we don't have the specialists available.
16. The doctors try their best, but never seem to prescribe enough medication or tell people things in plain language.
17. We can never get a bed in the local hospice when we need one
18. There's constant pressure to discharge patients early, which is inappropriate when you have dying patients on the ward.
19. I can't get the support I feel I need after a difficult death.
20. We can't seem to get the managers to recognise that death is something that happens frequently here, so there are no clear policies to deal with things.

These are anecdotal comments from practicing nurses, both students and qualified, representing heartfelt worries and concerns. They also reflect the complexity and competing demands of caring for the dying in both institutions and the home in the twenty-first century. It would be all too easy to dismiss such comments and to fall into the trap of the politically correct who would no doubt cite developments in clinical governance, supervision, audit, staff appraisal, autonomy, primary nursing, and care pathways as the answer to such anxieties.

While these developments have undoubtedly contributed to improved care and can empower staff in the right circumstances to force the agenda for the dying in their care, the daily reality for many clinical nursing staff remains overwhelmingly difficult.

This book could never present the reader with a universal panacea of answers for the twenty reasons cited above; indeed, it would be arrogant to assume as much, but it can and will challenge the reader to revisit this list and to review the merits of each statement as they use the good practice discussed within the text in their daily work.

How do we understand the real nature of palliative care and the nursing role?

To do that we need to make comparisons and to take account of how we normally view the world around us and the people in it.

The science perspective:

- sees the world as a complex form, full of facts, figures and definites
- views technology as aiding the working of society
- sees the world as fascinating, interesting and challenging in terms of research
- is more concerned with fact than feeling
- is underpinned by reason and logic
- proceeds by reason and law.

The art perspective:

- looks at the immediate appearance of the world
- takes account of the aesthetics and natural beauty of form
- values inspiration, imagination, creativity and intuition
- is more concerned with feeling than fact
- is underpinned by social and personal conscience
- proceeds by ethical and moral principles.

Looked at in this way, palliative care can rightly be said to be the combined whole experience of caring for people who are dying. It is an art and a science and this is a balance that is vital to the patient and the family. Ask yourself about the care that you give in your everyday practice. Is it dominated by procedures, routines, assessments and practical tasks (the science of caring)?

Or, is it dominated by a more psychological approach, involving the use of counselling techniques and therapeutic work in groups or with individuals (the art of caring)? Each is valid and we cannot expect to be skilled in all areas, but we can, and should, adopt a more balanced approach when the patient and family need it.

Perhaps one of the simplest ways of explaining this integration is to draw an analogy to an activity completely unrelated to nursing.

Motorcycling

Owning and riding a motorcycle is an experience that combines the art and the science of our perspective on the world. A motorcyclist needs to be aware of and understand some of the science of the machine in order to maintain it and ride it safely. They do not need to become a mechanic, but they do need to know how to adjust the chain where appropriate, and the suspension, set the tyre pressures, operate the controls, brake safely in different weather conditions and learn cornering technique. All this contributes to the science of motorcycling.

Once they begin riding the machine, the experience itself demands high concentration and psychomotor skills involving hands, feet, eyes and sometimes whole body movement. This is the science in action.

Very soon, however, the experience becomes one of practised and learnt skills which give pleasure and satisfaction to the rider. The visual appearance of the machine and its performance, handling and comfort give them confidence and enjoyment. As they develop their riding technique they learn to ride safer and quicker in different conditions. They use the science to enhance the art. The sense of freedom and control attained are arguably unique in motoring and the experience is based purely on the emotional and physical involvement in riding the motorcycle. This is the art and science acting in tandem, one is interdependent on the other.

There is a tendency today for people to think only in terms of one or the other. Medicine is dominated and ruled by the laws of science, which is perhaps why it is such an attractive profession and why it finds dealing with the art of care so difficult. Most of the other health professions aspire to the same ideals, nursing included. By doing this, they risk misunderstanding and underestimating the art of care, avoiding it because it gives little immediate satisfaction.

A motorcycle can be viewed as just a functional working collection of metal, plastics and fuel that sometimes breaks down. Just like our patients can be viewed as a biological entity which has gone wrong and needs medical intervention to put it right. However, just like nursing the dying person, when the motorcyclist takes the time to get to know the machine and begins to understand the way it behaves in different conditions and what makes it work, the journeys they make with it begin to become a shared experience. They find out what makes it unique and why it performs and behaves as it does. There are times when those journeys are difficult, tiring and challenging and they become very aware of their vulnerability and mortality; as a nurse sometimes feels when caring for the dying. It is at times like this that the significance of the journey becomes as important as the destination, as it is with our dying patients.

The quality of the rider's interaction with that motorcycle is proportional to the effort they alone put into the relationship they have with the machine. Similarly, the quality of a nurse's skill with the patients and relatives is directly proportional to the effort a nurse puts into balancing the science and the art of how they practice palliative care.

It is not the mechanics alone of the machine they ride that is important, its what they can achieve in the uniqueness of that relationship with that machine when they ride it that puts them in touch with the real heart and soul of motorcycling. It is logical and reasoned and at the same time an emotional and spiritual experience, just as caring for the dying, if done well, should be.

The challenge of delivering holistic palliative nursing care in the twenty-first century

A truly holistic approach involves valuing all the characteristics and past experience of the person. It demands an attitude and approach that goes beyond the diagnosis and immediate medical problem. Research clearly tells us that while control of physical pain is usually a priority for those who are dying, it is closely followed by concerns about the family and dependence (Rathbone *et al*, 1994; Maguire, 1995).

Achieving holistic care demands of the nurse a level of personal human contact with the dying person that goes beyond the tasks and procedures which can so often dominate everyday work.

Palliative care is the active total experience of caring for people who are dying. It is both a science and an art which is practised by a multi-professional team and emphasises normality and quality of life.

It values the whole person, and addresses their physical pain and discomfort, but also their feelings, their behaviours, their social issues, and their family and friends.

It is shaped by the individual's search for a sense of meaning and their desire for honesty, control over their life, and a need to maintain personal dignity as they see it, for the life they have left.

It is a combination of knowledge, skills and compassion in equal measure, that is both sensitive, hopeful, meaningful and dynamic. It is a way of thinking and an attitude of mind that should influence a nurse's behaviour whenever they work with a dying person in whatever setting.

References

Benner P (1984) F*rom Novice to Expert: Excellence and Power in clinical Practice*. California. Addison Wesley, California

Brown L (1986) The experience of care. Patient perspectives. *Top Clin Nurs* **8**(2): 56–62

Corner J, Bredin M, Krishnasamy M, Plant H (1999) Multi-centre randomised controlled trial of nursing intervention for breathlessness in patients with lung cancer. *Br Med J* **7188**(318): 901–4

European Association of Palliative Care (1989) *European Association of Palliative Care by Laws*. EAPC National Cancer Institute, Milan

Forest D (1989) The experience of caring. *J Adv Nurs* **14**: 815–13

Henderson V (1997) *Basic Principles of Nursing Care*. International Council of Nurses

Heslin K, Bramwell L (1989) The supportive role of the staff nurse in the hospital palliative care situation. *J Palliative Care* **5**: 20–6

Hinds PS, Martin J, Vogel RJ (1987) Nursing strategies to influence adolescent hopefulness during oncological illness. *J Associated Paediatric Nurses* **4**(2): 14–22

Kearney N (1999) New strategies in the management of cancer. *Cancer Nurs* **22**(1): 28–32

Macpherson G, ed (1992) *Blacks Medical Dictionary*. 37th edn. A & C Black, London: 434

Macintosh C, Bowles S (1997) Evaluation of a nurse-led acute pain service. *J Adv Nurs* **25**: 30–7

Maguire P (1995) Barriers top psychological care of the dying. *Br Med J* **291**: 1711–13

Manley K (1988) The needs and support of relatives. *Nursing* **3**(32): 19–22

Mayeroff M (1990) *On Caring*. 2nd edn. Harper Perennial, New York

Morse J, Bottorf J Neander W, Solberg S (1991) Comparative analysis of conceptualisation of caring. *Image J Nurse Sch* **23**(2): 119–26

National Council for Hospice and Specialist Palliative Care Services (1995) *Specialist Palliative Care: A Statement of Definitions*. Occasional Paper 8 NCHSPCA,

National Council for Hospice and Specialist Palliative Care Services (2001) *What do we mean by palliative care*. Discussion paper. No 9. NCHSPCA,

Patient Centred Cancer Services (1996) *What Patients Say*. The National Cancer Alliance. Oxford

Rathbone G, Horsley S, Goacher J (1994) A self-evaluated assessment for seriously ill hospice patients. *Palliative Med* **8**: 29–34

Reiman D (1986) Non-caring and caring in the clinical setting: Patients' perceptions. *Top Clin Nurs* **8**(2): 30–6

Roach M (1987) *The Human act of Caring: A Blueprint for the Health Professions*. Canadian Hospital Association, Ottowa

Smith MC, Sttullenbarger E (1995) An integrative review of oncology nursing research. 1981–91. *Cancer Nurs* **18**: 167–79

Taylor B, Glass N McFarlane J, Stirling C (1997) Palliative nurses' perceptions of the nature and effects of their work. *Int J Palliative Nurs* **3**(5): 253–8

Watson J (1985) *Nursing: The Philosophy and Science of Caring*. Colorado Associated Press, Boulder.

World Health Organization (1990) *Report of the WHO expert committee Geneva: Cancer Pain Relief and Palliative Care*. Technical Report Series 804

World Health Organization (2002) *National Cancer Control Programmes: Policies and Managerial Guidelines*, 2nd edn. WHO, Geneva

Useful websites

WHO link to: An exploration of the meaning of dignity in palliative care.
http://www.ejpc.co.uk/ejpc/ejpc5no6.htm

http://www.acsu.buffalo.edu/~drstall/dignity.txt

Oregon Death with Dignity Act May Improve End-Of-Life Care
http://www.medscape.com/Medscape/features/ResourceCenter/Hospice/public/R
    C-index-Hospice.html

Chapter links to the Nursing and Midwifery Council's (NMC's) *Code of Professional Conduct* (2002)

2. Respect the patient or client as an individual
    2.1 Partnership in care
    2.2 Promote and respect dignity

3. Obtain consent before you give any treatment or care
    3.1 The right to information
    3.2 Respect for autonomy

4. Cooperate with others in the team
    4.1 Defining the team members
    4.3 Communicate your skill, knowledge and expertise
    4.4 Ensure accurate record keeping

5. Protect confidential information
    5.1 Respect the use of information and guard against breaches of
        confidentiality
    5.2 Seek patient's wishes to share information

6. Maintain your professional knowledge and competence
    6.4 Facilitate the learning of others
    6.5 Deliver care based on evidence, research and best practice

Chapter 2

Encountering death for the first time

> You don't die in hospital any more you just achieve zero
> transitional probability to a higher state!

Junior doctor talking to a new student nurse on her first day on the ward.

There are some events in life that are truly formative experiences. Events that have a profound impact on us and can shape our values, attitudes and beliefs for the future. Being at the bedside of someone who is dying and being surrounded by the intensity of emotions, thoughts and behaviours exhibited is one such life experience. Its impact on a nurse meeting this for the first time can be profound and the memory remains fresh for a long time.

If you would like to test this statement then please take up this small challenge. The next time you go on duty and the moment is appropriate ask an experienced nurse to recall when she was first introduced to death in the clinical situation. You are likely to hear a story in such detail it may have occurred the previous week, rather than perhaps a decade or two ago. Reflective memories such as this are immensely powerful and can serve as useful learning tool for others.

Where and how do people die?

As a student nurse you will encounter a range of deaths in many different circumstances, however, the vast majority are likely to be expected deaths. At the beginning of the twentieth century most people died at home simply because there was no other option. Today, in our increasingly urban environment, some 60%–70% of people die in a hospital environment and only about 23–25 % in their own homes. Deaths in specialist environments account for about 3% due to the low overall number of beds, and deaths in the nursing home sector account for some 12%–15% with regional variations (Clarke, 1993).

What happens?

There are many physical changes in dying which are quite normal and usually do not cause discomfort. Dying patients will manifest some or all of the following:

- profound weakness
- difficulty swallowing, eg. medications
- the skin may turn pale, darker, blue, purple, patchy
- the body temperature may fall, or in some cases rise
- blood pressure is lower and may be harder to measure
- the sensation of being cold or hot may be lost.
- appetite may be lost
- the eyes may glaze over, not blink, stay open, or not see
- the mouth may be dry
- urine flow may stop or be dark
- control of bowels and bladder may be lost
- breathing may be irregular
- fluid in the lungs may cause a snoring type sound
- there may be more sleepiness and weakness (cannot speak or raise the hand)
- the sense of hearing (and possibly touch) are the last to go.

The signs of imminent death:

- patient cannot be easily roused
- patient stops breathing
- death is usually peaceful, not loud or violent
- profound skin pallor develops within half an hour of death.

Death is evident when there is no pulse, blood pressure, breathing and brain function for several minutes, and the pupils of the eyes stay wide open and do not change.

To gain a better idea of your first encounter with death please read this short extract from a published clinical article and reflect on the questions it poses.

James' mouth was partially open, his breathing erratic and laboured. His emaciated and jaundiced face resembled a wax-work figure in the dim light of the side ward. James lay motionless, his body showing vivid signs of the battle he had undergone against his terminal liver cancer. I sat quietly. but not at ease, watching every rise and fall of his chest. James had suffered for many weeks. He had grown close to all the staff in the ward during his illness and had requested to die here as he had no family and his friends lived far away. Tonight it was my turn to try and offer him comfort and support, during the long, quiet hours of the night shift. I pondered the meaning and significance of life, which at times seems so unfair. My attention turned to James. What was he feeling as he approached the end of his life? I started to think about my own end. How and when would that happen? I suddenly felt very cold and alone. I was brought back to the present when James' hand gently squeezed mine and he gave a shallow sigh. Then his breathing ceased and he lay still. The expression on his face had changed to one of peace and contentment. Death had visited the side ward not as an enemy, but as a friend.

McSherry W, 1996

Questions

1. Pick out some of the key words and phrases that made an impact on you when reading this story?
2. Now write down a few words or phrases that describe how you personally felt immediately after reading this story?

Consider:

⌘ Was it difficult to write down how you felt?
⌘ When do you think that you will encounter death for the first time as a student nurse?

How can I help? Your responsibilities

Some of the key nursing strategies that can be used to support patients and relatives when death is imminent are discussed by Becker (2001) and include:

⌘ **Spend time with dying patients**. It is all too easy to avoid the dying patient and their relative. Sometimes they need to be left alone, but there are many times when the need for human contact, comfort and reassurance is vital. The caring concept of 'being available' is acknowledged by a number of authors. It is synonymous with Parse's (1992) concept of 'True Presence' and is one of the carative factors used by Watson (1985). Benner and Wrubel (1989) note that:

The ability to presence oneself, to be with a patient in a way that acknowledges your shared humanity, is the basis of nursing as a caring practice.

⌘ **Answer questions.** A patient may ask a nurse, doctor or any member of the caring team, at any time, questions about their prognosis and diagnosis. They may also wish to discuss their thoughts and feelings surrounding this. All members of the direct caring team should have up-to-date knowledge about a patient's condition and should be prepared to share this if requested. There is much anxiety expressed by practicing nurses about this area, but there is no code, or rule, or law, which forbids a nurse to give this information if, in their judgement, it is the right thing to do at the time. The NMC's *Code of Professional Conduct* (2002) fully endorses this stance. For more information about techniques to use see *Chapter 8* on communication.

⌘ **Allow the patient to die.** This may sound rather obvious, but one of the major challenges of palliative nursing in non-specialist environments is empowering staff to reach a considered decision regarding the care orientation of the patient. Ideally, this should be done in conjunction with the patient, if possible, the relatives, and all members of the team. Much distress can be caused if efforts to initiate resuscitation or other procedures are fruitless, when the quality of the remaining life is poor. It is the simple ethical principle of 'non-maleficience' or, in other words, we should do the patient no harm. It requires an assertive and knowledgeable nurse who has a good understanding of accountability and confidence to challenge the *status quo* where necessary, if the patient's best interest is to be served.

⌘ **Understand the family.** It is good practice to assign a member of staff to discover what family there is, how they wish to be involved in care and what, if any, special needs they may have. This is not only part of the admission procedure, but a continuing responsibility thereafter, as relationships change and staff come and go. Although difficult to achieve, in some clinical environments, the sense of continuity achieved by this approach is highly valued by both patient and relatives.

⌘ **Consider where best to care for the dying person.** This decision will largely depend on the wishes of the patient and the family and their particular needs. Careful attention to the environment can provide good psychological support, by creating a milieu in which the patient is comfortable. Some patients may prefer peace and quiet and wish to be in a side room. Others, however, like to be part of life on a ward. Some may like to be moved closer to the office or staff desk. Such choice may not be available within the nursing and residential home, but the opportunity to personalise care within that environment is usually better due to greater continuity in staff and more long-term relationships. Those that die at home can have a wide variety of services to support them (depending on diagnosis unfortunately), but the psychological comfort of being in familiar surroundings is a powerful element. The key word to consider is choice.

⌘ **Respect the patient's interpretation of their dignity**. Don't build yourself a set of beliefs and values which unconsciously communicate to the patient and family that their loved one's death should represent an ideal. This can rarely be achieved in any environment, and is perhaps more often achieved at home or in a hospice. Let the patient decide what their priorities are and work towards these. Many people die with unfinished business in relationships and personal difficulties; this does not negate or devalue the care that has been given. We must learn to evaluate care based on what we know of the patient's values and beliefs and not our own.

The least you need to know

⌘ **Support:** Tell staff that this is your first experience and ask for help. Problems often occur simply because staff assume that you have experience in this area, as you appear confident, or because you are afraid to ask as you don't wish to appear incompetent. The good news is that your honesty will almost always be rewarded by being mentored by a nurse who is interested and sensitive.

⌘ **Sensitive:** Be aware that this is a unique occasion and not only will the relatives feel vulnerable but also yourself. You are being asked to step into and be part of one of life's most sensitive events. The family and friends around that bedside will consider you the expert, even though you are not. They have a right for a professional and caring approach which embraces both the science and art of palliative nursing (*Chapter 1*). This means that you may well feel upset, and on occasions demonstrate this by shedding a tear, or perhaps hugging a family member. Rest assured that this is no contradiction to professional practice, it does in fact enhance it .

⌘ **Talk:** Be sure to find a trusted person to talk to about it afterwards. If you have a mentor, or other such person available, use them for this purpose. It is important that your perceptions are shared and shaped in this way, so that good practice can be valued and potential issues addressed early on. If no such person is available at work then seek out a good friend or relative who can give you some quality time soon after.

⌘ **Alone:** If it is avoidable, no patient should die alone. There are always occasions when this is unavoidable, such as when someone lives alone, or during the night, or even when they are in the toilet in a busy hospital environment. There are numerous times, however, when a death is anticipated and expected. When this is the case no person should, unless they request it, be allowed to die alone. This is a clear nursing responsibility and should be taken seriously wherever dying takes place.

⌘ **Time:** Give yourself time to reflect on the significance of this event and how it has shaped your thinking. Reflective learning is not only an essential part of professional development, it also allows us to validate and gain a sense of perspective about what took place.

References

Becker R (2001) How will I cope: psychological aspects of advanced illness. In: Gamlin R, Kinghorn S, eds. *Palliative Nursing: Bringing comfort and hope*. Baillière Tindall, Edinburgh: chap 12

Benner P, Wrubel J (1989) *The Primacy of Care*. Addison Wesley, California

Clarke D, ed (1993) *The Future of Palliative Care: Issues of policy and practice*. Open University Press, Buckingham

Nursing and Midwifery Council (2002) *Code of Professional Conduct*. NMC, London

Parse RR (1992) Human becoming: Parse's theory of nursing. *Nurs Science Q* **5**: 35–42

McSherry W (1996) Reflections from a side ward. *Nurs Times* **92**(33): 29–31

Watson M (1994) Psychological care for cancer patients and their families. *J Ment Health* **3**: 457–65

Chapter links to the NMC's *Code of Professional Conduct* (2002)

2. Respect the patient or client as an individual
   2.2 Promote and respect dignity

3. Obtain consent before you give any treatment or care
   3.1 The right to information
   3.2 Respect for autonomy

6. Maintain your professional knowledge and competence
   6.1 Participate in regular learning activities

8. Act to identify and minimise the risk to patient's and clients
   8.1 promote a safe and therapeutic environment

Chapter 3

Palliative nursing skills: what are they?

Student:	*I think I'm a good listener.*
Clinical mentor:	*You're not as good at listening to patients as you think you are. I've noticed that you are frightened of silence. You need to practice this more.*
Student:	*It hurts a little to admit it, but you're right. I never realised.*

Just how competent are you to practice and how do you know that the skills you have developed are based around a sound evidence base. The issue of grading competency to practice in pre-registration nursing programmes is straightforward. The clinical assessor in the majority of instances is simply required to make a judgement, which indicates yes or no against a given statement. It can be legitimately argued that for the protection of the public, absolutes such as this are necessary. Yet the objectivity of such judgements is as much open to question as any other system.

Clearly with qualified nurses a different approach is needed. Work from people like Benner (1984) who saw nurses moving from 'novice to expert' on a continuum, provides us with a much clearer idea of the ways in which adults learn nursing in the 'real world' of practice, and relates closely to Carpers' (1978) four patterns of knowing, which she suggests should be present in each nursing act, ie:

- empirical knowledge
- aesthetic knowledge
- personal knowledge
- ethical knowledge.

The assessment tool used in this chapter, designed by Becker (2000), and the criteria by which you can assess your skills reflects the work of both these authors. For the majority of nurses, assessment of clinical skills is predominantly self-judgement validated by educators and only occasionally nurses in practice. This assessment usually takes the form of:

- reflective essays, diaries and journals
- portfolio development

- critical incident analysis
- learning contracts.

These are all familiar strategies and this kind of reflective process-centered assessment is very useful, but the ability to think and write effectively at a given academic standard does not necessarily translate into competence in clinical skills.

The tool is designed to be a means by which you can obtain a baseline assessment of your clinical skills development in using the palliative care approach wherever you work. It will help you to identify deficits in areas that need to be addressed, and to acknowledge skills that are already well developed. There is a simple, graduated scale used to enable you to make your decision as you work your way through the document.

What is in it?

There are a number of clearly written competency statements which are divided into six separate sections, each with a particular focus.

1   Communication skills.
2   Psychosocial skills.
3   Team skills.
4   Physical care skills.
5   Life closure skills.
6   Intrapersonal skills.

These areas have been shown by research (Davies and Oberle, 1990; Degner *et al*, 1991; Heslin and Bramwell, 1989; Taylor *et al*, 1997) to be the most representative of the true nature of palliative nursing. To help your understanding, a working definition of each of these areas is offered:

Explored:	To examine and investigate systematically an area or skill related to practice.
Practiced:	To take a skill and use it appropriately in the clinical area on a repeated basis.
Developed:	To progress in the knowledge, application and evaluation of a skill and demonstrate this in practice.

What is a competency

Generally speaking, competence in a given set of skills is based around the achievement of a desired standard of behaviour and expressed critical thinking. In order to work it relies on the formulation of agreed set competencies that are identified at differing levels of practice.

Sounds good in theory, but the reality can be somewhat more difficult to interpret.

What do I have to do ?

1. Read the competency document thoroughly and familiarise yourself with the competency statements and grading structure.
2. Set some time aside to conduct your own self-assessment of your current skills level as indicated in the document. This will help you to identify areas for development, which can be addressed in your clinical practice.
3. It is helpful if you can select between five to ten competencies that are priorities and these can then be written into a learning contract to help you focus on what needs to be done to move your skills forward. You may also wish to seek the opinion of a clinical mentor or trusted colleague who can assist you. You will find there are often clear areas of general agreement and some areas of disagreement — this is to be expected. The real learning and development rests upon your ability to examine the deficits and plan a strategy to deal with these issues in your everyday practice.
4. This tool also has the added advantage of clarifying and validating, where it is evident, what you perceive you are already competent at. This is equally important to our professional development as sometimes it can be difficult to acknowledge and articulate what we are good at, when it appears that the focus within the culture of nursing is centered upon being critical in the sense of poorly delivered care.
5. It is advantageous if the mentor you choose already knows something about you as a practicing nurse. They will be in a far better position to discuss your grading honestly with you.

The success of this approach lies very much in your ability to be both honest and reflective in your assessment. It is undoubtedly challenging, both intellectually and personally, to put one's perceived skills so closely under scrutiny, but if we are to improve the care of the dying in whatever setting it takes place, it is important to define clearly what it is we expect a nurse to be able to do, at what standard, and to empower them to be able to move practice forward. The evidence base presented by this competency tool is but one small step in this direction and is offered as an opportunity to engage in such work. It has been extensively evaluated in practice, peer reviewed, published and developed over several years.

Competency assessment document			
1. **Communication skills:** This refers to the range of interpersonal and counselling strategies used by the nurse with the patient and family members, and alludes to the truly empathic nature of the nurses' experience in a palliative care setting	**Self-assessment**		
	Explored	Practiced	Developed
Establishing a relationship: The nurse is able to: introduce herself, explain her role and obtain baseline biographical and illness related information.	☐	☐	☐
Use knowledge of verbal and non-verbal communication skills to spend time and establish a rapport with the patient and/or significant others to enable trust to develop.	☐	☐	☐
Building and maintaining a relationship: The nurse is able to:			
Spend time with the patient and family listening to their concerns and worries, respecting their beliefs and opinions in a climate of confidentiality.	☐	☐	☐
Use the skills of empathy and reflective questioning to enable the patient and family to talk freely if they wish to.	☐	☐	☐
Demonstrate a warm empathic, giving response when appropriate to communicate trust and understanding.	☐	☐	☐
Actively use the skills of facilitation and reflection to enable individuals to see each other's viewpoints in a supportive non-threatening environment.	☐	☐	☐
Professional relationships: The nurse is able to:			
Communicate key issues of relevance to the patient's care truthfully and unambiguously to the other members of the team.	☐	☐	☐
Articulate the ethical and moral reasoning behind nursing care decisions.	☐	☐	☐
Dealing with emotions: The nurse is able to:			
Recognise the context of expressed anger from patients and family as a valid emotion and to react calmly using active listening skills to defuse the situation.	☐	☐	☐
React professionally and objectively in a conflict scenario and use the other members of the team for guidance, support, and constructive reflection.	☐	☐	☐

Competency assessment document

2. Psychosocial skills: This is focused on a range of holistic skills which combine to enhance and support quality of life for the patient and family and help them to exercise choices in care and to come to terms with the impending loss.

Self-assessment

	Explored	Practiced	Developed

Philosophy of care: The nurse is able to:

	Explored	Practiced	Developed
Describe and accept the caring palliative concept of care as opposed to curative care.	☐	☐	☐
Accept that the person is dying and not feel guilty about being unable to stop the dying process.	☐	☐	☐

Facilitating: The nurse is able to:

	Explored	Practiced	Developed
Work with the patient and family helping them to plan strategies and offering options for palliative/terminal care and recognising and accepting others' limitations.	☐	☐	☐
Inspire trust and confidence in the dying patient and family by the use of 'self' in the clinical situation.	☐	☐	☐
Structure one's time effectively so as to create opportunities for spontaneity in the life of the dying person.	☐	☐	☐
Recognise and acknowledge the patient's unique personal abilities, giving approval, supporting choices, and providing a realistically hopeful environment within the patient's limitations.	☐	☐	☐

Finding meaning: The nurse is able to:

	Explored	Practiced	Developed
Accept the beliefs and values of others, although they may differ widely from his/her own.	☐	☐	☐
Show an awareness and understanding of the beliefs, attitudes and practices of other cultural and ethnic groups within our society.	☐	☐	☐
Help patients make sense of their illness and prognosis by offering hope, facilitating reflection of life and values, fulfilling their wishes and attempting to meet spiritual needs.	☐	☐	☐
Use sensitive judgement to talk openly about death, where appropriate, when patients and families want to do so.	☐	☐	☐
Help the patient to come to terms with the idea of their own mortality and impending death in a supportive empathic environment.	☐	☐	☐

Competency assessment document

3. Team skills: This area acknowledges the interdisciplinary nature of palliative care and the need to liaise actively with other disciplines on the patient's behalf.

Self-assessment

	Explored	Practiced	Developed
Advise the team on a range of possible options to help alleviate the patient's and family's distress.	☐	☐	☐
Demonstrate that they can negotiate the health care system on behalf of the patient and family by sharing and consulting with other team members.	☐	☐	☐
Mentor and support students in the practice of palliative care.	☐	☐	☐
Work as an equal member of the multidisciplinary team and assert the needs and rights of the patient and family when needed.	☐	☐	☐
Recognise the need for emotional support with colleagues and provide this, where appropriate, in a trusting, confidential manner.	☐	☐	☐

4. Physical care skills: This area is about the knowledge and skills necessary for the delivery of active, hands-on care in whatever setting.

Controlling pain and symptoms: The nurse is able to:

	Explored	Practiced	Developed
Demonstrate and articulate an active commitment to the relief of pain and the palliation of distressing symptoms.	☐	☐	☐
Discuss the concept of total pain and the need for a holistic approach to the assessment of pain.	☐	☐	☐
Use effectively the pain assessment tools available in their clinical area and regularly review the assessment.	☐	☐	☐
Show competency in the assessment of total pain.	☐	☐	☐
Demonstrate a sound knowledge of the WHO analgesic ladder and discuss the appropriate use of opiates and adjuvant therapies.	☐	☐	☐
Describe the means by which oral opiate doses are calculated for administration subcutaneously.	☐	☐	☐
Provide a rationale for the use of a syringe driver in the palliation of pain, nausea and vomiting, restlessness and agitation.	☐	☐	☐
Recognise situations where psychological therapies and spiritual support can be of benefit to the patient in the assessment and control of total pain.	☐	☐	☐
Organise the administration of medication, regularly reviewing the situation, anticipating possible problems and reacting to presenting problems.	☐	☐	☐
Advise the patient and family where appropriate, on the range of possible options to help alleviate current symptomatology.	☐	☐	☐
Teach and explain about medication dosages, changes in care and enable the patient and family to understand what is happening to them, to strengthen their ability to do things for themselves.	☐	☐	☐

Competency assessment document

5. Life closure skills: This area is concerned with nursing behaviours, which are crucial to the dignity of the patient and family as they perceive it when life is close to an end, and thereafter.

Self-assessment

Explored   Practiced   Developed

Maintaining a sense of calm: The nurse will be able to:

Foster an environment of peace and family involvement in care where appropriate by attempting to control factors such as noise, privacy and interruptions.

☐   ☐   ☐

At the bedside: The nurse will be able to:

Discuss the fact of imminent death with family members of the dying person.

☐   ☐   ☐

Notify families where deterioration is taking place, and make provision for family comfort throughout.

☐   ☐   ☐

Judge when to defer physical care when death is approaching.

Encourage family members to sit close to the dying person and maintain touch and conversation where possible.

☐   ☐   ☐

Explain the signs of impending death to the family, where appropriate, and with sensitivity.

☐   ☐   ☐

After death: The nurse will be able to :

☐   ☐   ☐

Provide the family with the time, space and privacy to stay with the deceased for as long as they wish and encourage them to say goodbye and express their feelings.

☐   ☐   ☐

Competency assessment document

6. Intrapersonal skills: This refers to a nurse's philosophical understanding of the true nature of palliative nursing and alludes to the ability to maintain self-esteem and self-worth by acknowledging and questioning personal behaviours and feelings as an integral part of effective functioning.

Self-assessment

	Explored	Practiced	Developed
Global values: The nurse will be able to:			
Demonstrate respect for the inherent worth of others, coupled with a predisposition to look for the good things in people, and an intrinsic belief in this.	☐	☐	☐
Particular values: The nurse will be able to:			
Show a developed understanding of an individual's unique characteristics and abilities which occurs over time and is reflective in nature and presentation.	☐	☐	☐
Recognise their own skill and competence in caring for a dying person and seeks to improve these skills and knowledge in themselves and other members of the care team.	☐	☐	☐
Self-oriented values: The nurse will be able to:			
Be genuine, open and honest in interactions with the patients, family and colleagues.	☐	☐	☐
Accept and acknowledge compliments and feedback from a variety of sources, which reinforce the value of the nurse's contribution to care.	☐	☐	☐
Looking inward: The nurse will be able to:			
Discuss and reflect periodically on the meaning and significance of life and death events in relation to work by drawing on insights and spiritual awareness.	☐	☐	☐
Deal introspectively with his/her own reactions to loss and utilise past experience in interactions with individuals facing impending or actual loss.	☐	☐	☐
Acknowledging own reaction: The nurse will be able to:			
Recognise and attempt to understand their own reactions and feelings when nursing the dying and bereaved, reflecting on how this affects the care given in sensitive situations.	☐	☐	☐

Suggested learning contract

Identified competency: ------------------------------------

Self-assessment rating:

Explored ☐   Practiced ☐   Developed ☐

Resources and strategies: (what do I need to do to improve my competency level?)

Evidence of accomplishment: (How can I demonstrate what I have learnt?)

Target date: ------------------------------------

Criteria for validating skills accomplishment`:

How do you now judge your skill in this competency?

Explored ☐   Practiced ☐   Developed ☐

How does your clinical mentor/trusted colleague judge your skill in this competency?

Explored ☐   Practiced ☐   Developed ☐

The least you need to know

⌘ Read the competency document thoroughly and familiarise yourself with the competency statements and grading structure.

⌘ Set some time aside to conduct your own self-assessment of your current skills level as indicated in the document.

⌘ Truly meaningful assessment of your clinical skills requires a mature level of honesty and self-insight.

⌘ Be good to yourself and acknowledge the positive level of skills you already have.

Supportive references

Becker R (2000) Competency assessment in palliative nursing. *Eur J Palliative Care* **7**(3): 88–91

Benner P (1984) *From Novice to Expert: Excellence and power in clinical practice*. Addison Wesley, California

Carper B (1978) Fundamental patterns of knowing in nursing. *Adv Nurs Sci* **1**(v): 1323

Davies B, Oberle K (1990) Dimensions of the supportive role of the nurse in palliative care. *Oncol Nurs Forum* **17**(1): 87–94

Degner LF, Gow CM, Thompson LA (1991) Critical nursing behaviours in care for the dying. *Cancer Nurs* **14**(5): 246–53

Heslin K, Bramwell L (1989) The supportive role of the staff nurse in the hospital palliative care situation. *J Palliative Care* **5**: 20–6

Taylor B, Glass N, McFarlane J, Stirling C (1997) Palliative nurses' perceptions of the nature and effects of their work. *Int J Palliative Nurs* **3**(5): 253–8

Useful websites

Royal College of Nursing — go to specialist palliative care competencies project
http://www.rcn.org.uk/members/publications/

Chapter links to the NMC's *Code of Professional Conduct* (2002)

6. Maintain your professional knowledge and competence
    6.1 Participate in regular learning activities
    6.2 Acknowledge the limits of your competence
    6.3 Obtain help to develop skills and competence

Chapter 4

Pain and suffering in advanced illness

My name is Graham, I have advanced cancer. At first there was no pain now it hurts everywhere. They give me lots of medicines but don't seem to understand how much death and leaving loved ones hurts. Very soon I will be a pile of ashes. Please try to understand, this is what hurts most.

Definitions of pain

Pain has been defined in many ways. The International Association for the Study of Pain (IASP 1986) described it as:

> *An unpleasant sensory and emotional experience associated with actual or potential tissue damage, or described in terms of such damage.*

Melzack and Wall (1982) describe pain as a 'category of complex experiences not a single sensation produced by a single stimulus'. Most qualified nurses and students are able to quote McCaffery (1972) who said, 'Pain is what the experiencing person says it is, existing whenever he says it does'. Pain is a highly subjective experience. No two patients' experience will be the same. It is mere rhetoric to quote McCaffery and then go on to question the validity of the patient's account of their pain. If we are to treat pain effectively patients **must** be allowed to give an account of their pain and they **must** be believed.

Types of pain

Pain is divided into two main types: nociceptive and neuropathic. All over the body there are sensory organs in the tips of nerves which detect pain. They are called nociceptors. They transmit nerve impulses via the spinal cord to the brain. The frequency and intensity of these impulses tell us where the pain is and how severe it is. When stimulated they evoke a reflex action like when we touch something hot.

Neuropathic pain arises when nerves which carry messages of sensation including pain, light, touch, vibration, warmth and coldness are compressed or damaged by disease or an accident. The pain is then felt in the area of the body supplied by that nerve. An example of this is when the Herpes Zoster virus becomes active, as in shingles. Severe pain is felt in blisters arising in the nerve's territory and the pain can persist long after the skin has healed.

Suffering

It is difficult to reduce suffering to a simple definition. Even when pain is well controlled patients can suffer. In life we hope to find peace, love and understanding, wholeness and meaning. Knowing that one is dying, saying goodbye to loved ones, friends who don't visit, losing the ability to walk, enjoy food, make love all contribute to suffering; yet the extremes of human deprivation and the crucible of terminal illness teach us that, even in the direst circumstances, peace is possible (Mount, 2003).

Staff who care for the dying may suffer too. Students sometimes feel this more acutely than qualified colleagues who have developed a social structure and shared coping mechanisms. Students can feel a sense of 'failure', 'I didn't know what to say', 'I didn't know what to do'. They experience anger, guilt and loss of control. They don't feel involved in decision making and may be excluded from social events, supervision or post-death review meetings.

Staff who constantly work with dying patients are exposed to serious illness, disability, loss, pain and death. They stare suffering in the face. Students also suffer as they go from one placement to another without the chance to integrate fully into the team. If suffering is not acknowledged, this can lead to exhaustion and damaged relationships.

Quality of life and a sense of being healthy do not correlate with a sense of well being. It is possible to experience profound physical disability and, at the same time, a high quality of life. Victor Frankl's wonderful book (1959) *Man's Search for Meaning* tells of his experiences while captive in a Nazi concentration camp. He concluded that our human quest is not for fame and fortune but for meaning. Meaning, he suggests, may be found in five domains:

1. Things created or accomplished.
2. Things left to others, to be remembered by.
3. Things we believe in.
4. Things loved.
5. The experience of suffering.

When hope of cure is no longer realistic, the above five domains serve as prompts for our conversations with the dying and bereaved. For example:

When you look back over your life, what are you most proud of?

What do you feel you will be remembered for?

Who and what have you loved?

Mother Theresa of Calcutta said: 'In this life we can not do great things. We can only do small things with great love.'

> **Tanya's story:**
>
> I recently returned to work as a community staff nurse having cared for a much loved relative at home up to his death. Do you know what support I received as I watched him die, every ounce of strength and humanity draining from his weakened body? **Nothing**. Do you know what support I received when I returned after what is laughingly known as 'compassionate leave' **Nothing**, Oh that's not true, the sister said, can you take Tanya's terminal's off her until she has had a chance to catch up with her paper work? Tanya's voice trembled, her eyes filled with tears of anger and disappointment.

Pain is a common experience

Think back over the last six months or so and make a note of any pain you have experienced. Your list will may contain some of the following: headache, back pain, toothache, period pain, arthritis, gastritis. You may have included pain that has a more psychological origin, such as the pain of losing a loved one through death, divorce or separation. From this simple exercise we can learn two important lessons.

- ⌘ In everyday life some degree of pain is common. Patients with cancer or other advancing illnesses frequently experience pain that is **not** due to their disease. These types of pain require as much attention as cancer pain.
- ⌘ Pain is not simply a physical phenomenon. Psychological and other factors affect the way we experience pain. Neglecting any of the contributing factors will result in poor pain control.

Incidence of pain in advanced illness

When we think of cancer we often think of pain, but one third of patients with cancer do not experience severe pain. The good news is that, of the two-thirds of cancer patients who do experience severe pain, most will have their pain adequately controlled by the application of basic principles of pain management. Of those cancer patients who have pain, 80% have more than two pains (Twycross and Lack, 1984).

Accurate assessment of each pain is the cornerstone of pain management as some pains in patients with advancing cancer are due to non-malignant causes — and different types of pain are treated differently. Patients with long-term pain problems that are not adequately controlled suffer both physically and mentally.

The concept of total pain

Look at the diagram representing total pain (*Figure 4.1*) (Saunders, 1967). This illustrates the complex and often interacting factors that influence the way we experience or perceive pain. A key point to remember is that medication can influence few of the contributing factors. Most, if not all, can be influenced by skilled nursing.

Assessing the patient in pain

Assessment is not a 'one-off' intervention, but part of a continuous process. Pain assessment is the foundation of pain management. Without it, pain cannot be controlled. Sudden, severe pain in patients with cancer is a medical emergency and patients must be assessed and treated without delay.

Begin your assessment by looking at the patient. Look for non-verbal cues that suggest pain, for example, body posture and facial expression. If your suspicion is aroused you may say something like, 'By the way you are sitting you look in pain?'

Much of your pain assessment will revolve around a series of questions. Questioning should take place in a conversational style rather than an interrogation. It is not essential to ask all questions in one 'sitting'. The aim of pain assessment is to gather as much information about the patient's pain as possible. Don't forget to ask all team members about the patient's pain. Professionals such as physiotherapists and social workers may have something to add. So, too, may the home support workers and domestic staff.

Suggested questions:

- ~ *Would you like to tell me about your pain?*
- ~ *What words do you use to describe your pain?*
- ~ *Can you show me where it hurts?*
- ~ *Is the pain there all the time?*
- ~ *How long have you had this pain?*
- ~ *Does the pain go anywhere else?*
- ~ *What makes the pain better?*
- ~ *What makes the pain worse?*
- ~ *What medications are you taking for the pain?*
- ~ *Do they help?*
- ~ *Are you taking them as your doctor prescribed? (If not, why not)?*
- ~ *Are you taking any medications your doctor did not prescribe, for example, ibuprofen you bought from the supermarket?*
- ~ *How do you feel about taking strong painkillers?*
- ~ *Is there anything else you would like to tell me about your pain?*

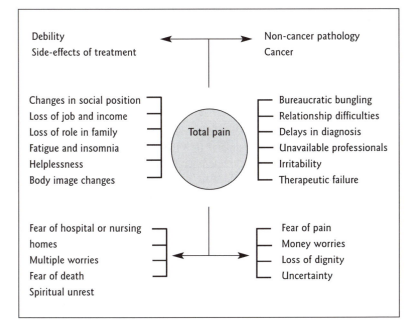

Figure 4.1: The concept of total pain (first described by Saunders, 1967)

For further information on pain assessment and other aspects of pain management see Gamlin and Lovel (2001).

Assessment tools and documentation

Many useful pain assessment tools exist. Tools must be simple to use for the patient and professional. (Don't go straight to the tools before you allow the patient to tell their story.) For further information on pain assessment tools see Farrar (2001).

Body outlines

These allow the user to indicate where the pain(s) is experienced. Ask the patient to show you where the pain(s) are.

Rating scales

```
                                                              10
   0  ─────────────────────────────────────────────  Worst pain
No pain                                                  imaginable
```

Ask the patient to give their pain a numerical or verbal rating. For example, a score out of ten with 0 = no pain and 10 = the worst pain imaginable. While these scales are helpful, please remember that pain is a highly subjective experience that is difficult to reduce to a number. Many patients find pain scales difficult to use.

Whatever tool and assessment approach is used it is essential that you record your findings for others to use. A seemingly insignificant comment may provide useful clues to your colleagues.

Pain diaries

Patients may find it useful to keep a diary about their pain. A simple format will suffice (*Figure 4.2*).

Keeping a diary can become tedious for some. For others, it

encourages them to focus on their pain. The main benefit is the record it provides to promote discussion about when the pain is worse and, more positively, what helps to alleviate pain.

Date	Time 0–5	Pain score	Activity	Comments
Monday	9.00	4	Getting ready	Hurts when I bend
Monday	9.45	2	Resting	Took morphine 10mg
Monday	11.40	1	Talked to GP	Really helped
Monday	13.00	5	Walking, windy day	Pain in face very bad Took pink medicine
Monday	15.00	0	Sleeping	
Monday	17.30	2	Eating tea	Pain behind breast bone

Case study: Peter

Peter is a forty-three-year-old man with advanced bowel cancer. His lower abdominal pain is well-controlled with morphine. While in the bathroom with Sam, a first-year student nurse, Peter says, 'I have a terrible pain down my right leg but I don't like to bother the doctors'. Sam asks a few questions and asks Peter to describe his pain. Peter says, 'It comes from nowhere like an electric shock down my leg'. 'I am terrified waiting for it to come back and I can't sleep'.

Sam passes this information on to Joe, the charge nurse. Together, they talk with Peter and then discuss Peter's pain with the doctors. They conclude that this is a neuropathic pain and Peter begins to take amitriptyline. Within a few days Peter's pain is much better and he is sleeping well.

More than one pain

Jack is a sixty-eight-year old man with advanced lung cancer. Sue, a second year student nurse assesses Jack's pain. At the ward meeting, attended by the multidisciplinary team, they draw the following conclusions about Jack's pain.

Low back pain due to bony secondaries in the lumbar spine. Headache due to worrying about his family. A burning pain in the right arm due to brachial plexus involvement. Pain due to arthritis in the left hip. Gastritis since he began taking Diclofenac.

Note that two out of the four pains are **not** caused by cancer and they will not all respond well to morphine.

Having listened to the patient's story and formed a picture of the pain consider what may be done to help.

The analgesic ladder (*Figure 4.3*) is a simple, reliable and effective way to understand pharmacological management of cancer pain. For a fascinating up-to-date review of the WHO analgesic ladder see Porta-Sales *et al* (2003).

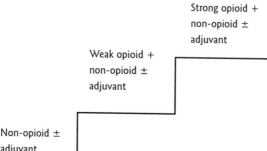

Figure 4.3: The World Health Organisation Analgesic Ladder (WHO, 1986, 1996)

All details about medication can be found in the *Palliative Care Formulary* (Twycross *et al*, 2002).

Step one

Patients are treated with non-opioid analgesics such as paracetamol, or non-steroidal anti-inflammatory drugs such as ibuprofen or Diclofenac (NSAIDs). Adverse effects such as gastric irritation and peptic ulceration are common with NSAIDs. Many patients will respond well to regular doses of step one drugs.

Step two

Patients with moderate pain, who are not pain-free on step one should be treated with a weak opioid drug, together with other drugs as necessary. Weak opioids include; codeine, dihydrocodeine and tramadol. You will be familiar with co-codamol, a mixture of paracetamol and codeine and co-dydramol which combines paracetamol and dihydrocodeine. These drugs are effective and very commonly prescribed. Their main drawback is the fixed combination of component drugs.

Step three

Patients experiencing severe pain or those who are not pain free on step two should receive a strong analgesic. If necessary, this can be combined with non-opioid drugs. Strong opioids include; morphine, diamorphine and fentanyl. Alternative opioids exist, for example, hydromorphone, methadone and oxycodone. It is essential to consult a pain specialist or palliative care specialist before prescribing alternative opioids.

When using analgesic drugs remember that the severity of pain, on its own does not give enough information to choose analgesics. Not every patient will require strong opioids. They should never be used as euphoriants or sedatives, ie. to elevate the mood or to sedate.

Not all pains are sensitive to opioids. If the pain is partially sensitive or not sensitive to opioids consider adjuvant or additional analgesics or other methods, such as trans-cutaneous electrical nerve stimulation (TENS). Nerve blocks or spinal procedures can be helpful. The advice of a palliative care specialist should be sought

It is important for the team to think about treatable cause of pain. For example, radiotherapy can be used to treat bone metastasis and surgery to fix a long bone that is about to fracture.

Morphine

Morphine is a highly effective and safe analgesic drug. Unfortunately, numerous morphine myths exist. Patients, their families and professionals often believe these myths, resulting in poor pain management.

Morphine myths

⌘ **Morphine is highly addictive:** Addiction is a psychological craving for a drug. It is defined only by psychological dependence, ie. compulsive use of a drug for its mood-altering properties, and continued use despite harm. This is very rare in cancer patients. Patients who 'appear' to be addicted, asking for another dose of medication, are usually still in pain. They, 'clock watch' desperate for the next dose to relieve their pain. Patients with a history of drug misuse can still be given opioid analgesics. A pain or palliative care specialist should be consulted for advice.

⌘ **Morphine will cause respiratory depression:** Again this is very rare. Pain itself is a strong respiratory stimulant. If respiratory depression occurs it can be managed with a drug called naloxone.

❧ **Patients will need more and more morphine as their disease progresses:** This is not usual. If patients do require escalating doses it is often a sign that the pain is not responding well to morphine or that other drugs or interventions are more appropriate

❧ **Morphine means this is the end:** Sadly, many patients believe this. It is understandable because most of the information they have received during their lives will have been negative. Some professionals also believe this and withhold morphine until the patient is near the end of life. At times, nurses blame doctors for not prescribing sufficient morphine. This may be true but nurses sometimes withhold medication that has been prescribed correctly, believing it to be harmful.

Morphine preparations

If at all possible, morphine should be given by mouth. It can be given as immediate release oral morphine solution or as a tablet. Morphine is effective for four hours, therefore it must be given every four hours, **not six- or eight-hourly**. There is not a standard dose for morphine. It is good practice to administer regular doses of oral morphine every four hours until the correct dose is established. This is known as dose titration.

Remembering to take a pain medication every four hours can be a burden. Morphine is also available in a preparation which is released over twelve hours; for example, MST or Zomorph and a twenty-four-hour preparation known as MXL.

There is rarely a place in palliative care for intra-muscular or intravenous injections. Intravenous injections of diamorphine are indicated if a patient has a myocardial infarction or, very occasionally, when severe pain is experienced. Intra-muscular injections are no more effective than subcutaneous injections and they are unpleasant particularly if the patient has lost a lot of weight.

Diamorphine

Chemically, diamorphine is very similar to morphine but it has one big advantage over morphine. It is very soluble, therefore it is suitable to be given by injection. Diamorphine may be given by regular subcutaneous injection. Often it is given using a syringe driver. This is a device driven by a battery which slowly and accurately injects medication from a syringe. This method is used when patients are unable to swallow or if they experience troublesome nausea. (For more information about using syringe drivers contact your specialist palliative care nurse.)

Fentanyl

Fentanyl is a powerful opioid analgesic. It is commonly administered intravenously during anaesthesia or in intensive therapy units. It is also available in a 'patch', worn on the skin like a sticking plaster. This method of drug delivery is well established as a method of delivering nicotine in people who wish to stop smoking and in hormone replacement therapy. Fentanyl is absorbed slowly through the skin. It is not effective immediately, therefore other opioids will continue to be given for a few hours. The patch needs to be changed every seventy-two hours. It is useful in patients who have achieved good pain control with other opioids. It is also suggested that patients using the fentanyl patch experience less constipation and are less sleepy during the day than patients taking morphine.

Adverse effects of opioids

These are well known. They are predictable and treatable. Simple clear explanations will do much to alleviate distress.

Constipation

Almost all patients receiving a mild or strong opioid will become constipated. This will remain an issue for the duration of treatment. Prescribing a regular prophylactic laxative with the opioid can prevent constipation. A combined stimulant and softener is appropriate.

Nausea and vomiting

One to two thirds of patients starting opioids will experience nausea. Within five to ten days most patients will feel better. They will benefit from prophylactic anti-emetic drugs. Low dose haloperidol is the drug of choice. Remember that, as well as opioid use, there are many possible causes for nausea in patients with advanced illness.

Sedation

Opioids and other drugs may cause sedation. Patients should be told of this side-effect. After a few days it tends to be less of a problem but the dose of drug(s) may need to be altered.

Dry mouth

Again, opioids and other drugs may cause this. Simple remedies such as frequent sips of a favourite drink will help as will good mouth care.

Less common side-effects include; hypotension, poor concentration, confusion, urinary hesitancy, itch and respiratory depression.

Pain is treated pharmacologically according to these principles:

- by the mouth — wherever possible
- by the clock — pain medications must be given regularly according to their known effects **so that the pain does not return**
- by the ladder – if a drug on the bottom step of the ladder is not easing the pain, move up a step of the ladder. A different drug on the same level is unlikely to be helpful.

The correct dose of analgesic is one which relieves the pain with minimum side-effects.

Other drugs used to manage pain

Although not thought of as analgesic drugs, other drugs can be used to manage pain in patients with advanced illness.

- ⌘ Antidepressant drugs: amitriptyline can be used to manage neuropathic pain. Given in small doses amitriptyline is not used to manage depression. It works by modifying the transmission of pain impulses.
- ⌘ Anticonvulsants: gabapentin (this is the only anticonvulsant licenced for pain control), carbamazepine, and sodium valproate and also modify pain impulses.
- ⌘ Antispamodics: hyoscine butylbromide relieves pain by reducing smooth muscle contraction. Particularly helpful in bowel colic.
- ⌘ Antispastics: are helpful in skeletal muscle tension in multiple sclerosis. Diazepam and other medications, such as baclofen have been used.
- ⌘ Corticosteroids: cortisone, prednisolone and dexamethasone work by reducing inflammation surrounding tumours.
- ⌘ Antibiotics: are highly effective in reducing pain due to inflammation when the cause is infective.

Breakthrough pain and incident pain

Regular doses of appropriate analgesia successfully manage pain in the majority of patients. Pain may return between regular doses particularly if the patient is mobile or having a dressing change. When taking opioids the dose for breakthrough pain is one sixth of the total prescribed twenty-four-hour dose. For example, a patient receiving 40mg of oral immediate release morphine every four hours has a total twenty-four-hour dose of 240mg. The breakthrough dose prescribed should be 40mg.

Other measures will help during painful procedures. Additional doses of analgesic drugs should be given well before a known painful procedure. Nurses should be sure that an intervention is really necessary before carrying it out. Entonox, a mixture of oxygen and nitrous oxide, may be helpful. You may be familiar with this used in childbirth. Check the procedure in your placement and ensure you understand how and when to use entonox.

Radiotherapy

Radiotherapy can be very effective to treat the pain caused by bone metastases. The patient may only require one or two treatments and may gain benefit within a few days

Trans-cutaneous electrical nerve stimulation (TENS)

This device has been used for many years to help in the management of different types of pain. It has proved useful in pain due to trapped nerves , ie. sciatica and for people who get phantom limb pain after an amputation. The TENS equipment consists of three parts; the stimulator, the leads and the electrodes. The stimulator is powered by a 9 volt battery. The electrodes are made of carbon rubber. They are placed, usually near the pain, and the stimulator is adjusted to create a feeling of gentle but strong stimulation in the skin. Sometimes pain relief is immediate while in some people it may take time to be effective. With TENS the patient is in control. TENS will not be effective in all types of pain but may be a useful addition to other approaches. Patients may be referred to a pain clinic for specialist advice.

Nerve blocks and spinal procedures

Although used infrequently, these procedures are valuable when complex or intractable pain exists. Local anaesthetic agents, opioids and other drugs are injected around nerves. One advantage is that small doses of opioids are used and side-effects are reduced. Some patients receiving local anaesthetic agents dislike the loss of sensation. Bowel and bladder function can be disturbed. The advice of an anaesthetist, pain or palliative care specialist is essential.

What else can be done to manage pain?

Analgesic drugs will always form the foundation of pain management in advanced illness, but we must not neglect other things that can help, for example:

- the help, advice and support of another professional such as a physiotherapist, occupational therapist, psychologist or social worker
- heat or cold
- a soak in a deep warm bath
- relaxation exercises
- someone to talk to
- someone who will listen but not judge when the patient is sad, angry or confused
- consideration of the emotional, psychological, social and spiritual aspects of pain
- distraction, for example, watching television or reading a book
- a gentle massage
- a comfortable bed and chair
- a good night's sleep
- an alcoholic drink
- good food and company.

Think about what you can do to facilitate the above. You may think that you do not have the skills to provide some of the comfort measures suggested. It is not necessary to attend a massage course to give a hand massage although you should not use aromatherapy products without permission. Massage and other comfort measures show that you have time and concern and put you in a place where you have time to listen and respond to worries and concerns. This, in itself, may help to reduce pain.

Relaxation techniques

Pain causes muscle tension and tense muscles ache causing more pain. Teaching simple relaxation exercises helps the patient to bring muscle tension under control and break the cycle. Relaxation and imagery are part of a repertoire of techniques which can bring comfort to the dying and bereaved

Benefits of relaxation

- reduction in autonomic activity
- lower pulse rate
- lower blood pressure
- lower temperature
- decreased muscular tension
- pain reduction
- aids rest and sleep
- feeling of well being
- feeling of control and mastery.

Relaxation methods

Relaxation methods aim to reduce tension by physical, psychological, spiritual or combined approaches. Like all skills, relaxation requires practice to become proficient. Ideally, patients would learn to relax in a quiet warm environment free of interruptions. These conditions are difficult to attain in real life and patients say they can learn to relax in the most challenging situations.

Progressive muscular relaxation

This is the easiest method to teach and to learn. The patient is guided through a sequence of simple and straightforward tensing and relaxing exercises so that he/she can become aware of the difference between tension and relaxation. It can begin with the patient tensing and relaxing hands and arms and then working from head to toe. It is important to know the patient in terms of his pain so that painful areas can be avoided.

Guided imagery or fantasy

Relaxing images are used to help the patient to divert his attention from where he is to an imaginary scene, such as a favourite holiday scene or a comforting image of home. The teacher can use his/her own images or make use of the patient's own images. Occasionally, patients find they are unable to see an image in their 'mind's eye'.

Autogenic relaxation

This method consists of a series of easy mental exercises designed to switch off the 'fight or flight' response in the body and replace it with a relaxation response. Autogenic relaxation is usually taught in a group over a series of weeks. Training consists of learning basic exercises which involves visualising particular instructions such as feelings of heaviness, warmth, and coolness in different parts of the body. It is claimed to be helpful in stress-related disorders. In palliative care, it can be adapted and taught in shorter sessions.

Hypnosis/hypnotherapy

The general public and some healthcare professionals sometimes think of hypnosis as something mystical and magic. Hypnotherapy aims to facilitate an altered state of consciousness in which the mind becomes very deeply relaxed. In such a state the patient is very susceptible to positive and beneficial suggestions. It has been used in palliative care where it has many practical applications, eg. pain management, management of symptoms such as nausea and vomiting, particularly anticipatory vomiting and dyspnoea, fear and anxiety management and phobia management. Hypnotherapy is a safe and effective approach but should only be used by those who have been specifically trained.

Meditation

Meditation is another approach to relaxation which requires the user to practice quiet relaxation. A mantra is used as a focus to deepen the relaxation. The mantra is usually a neutral sound without specific meaning which is repeated silently over and over again. This helps the user to concentrate thoughts inwardly and almost block out the outside world. Concentrating on objects such as a candle in a darkened room or a flower or pleasant odours form useful alternatives to the mantra. The patient with advanced illness is unlikely to be able to devote extended periods of time to meditation. Nevertheless, many patients may be able to deepen their relaxation by applying the principles of meditation.

Deep breathing

Teachers often ask their subjects to focus on their breathing or become aware of the breathing or notice their breathing. This is undoubtedly helpful for some patients but unhelpful for others. Approximately 50% of patients with advanced cancer have difficulty in breathing. Focusing on breathing may be helpful but conversely may cause distress. If in doubt, it may be better to avoid mentioning breathing.

You may have learned relaxation skills on placements such as maternity or mental health. After consulting with your qualified colleagues, consider their use in patients with advanced illness. Combine relaxation, where possible, with nursing measures such as bathing, wound care or when you notice a patient appears tense.

Conclusion

Pain, suffering and the fear of pain are terrible, but not inevitable consequences of cancer and other advancing illnesses. In this chapter we have seen that much can be done to relieve or help patients cope with their pain and suffering. Students of healthcare are in a privileged position because they play a vital role in assessing, planning, delivering and evaluating pain management.

Principles of cancer pain control (adapted from Regnard and Tempest, 1998)

- ❖ Pain may be due to: cancer, treatment and pathology other than cancer
- ❖ Ensure the entire team has adequate skills and knowledge
- ❖ Communicate all pain-related findings to the team
- ❖ Observe patients carefully. Don't wait for them to tell you they have pain
- ❖ Assess pain meticulously and repeatedly
- ❖ Monitor the effectiveness of pain relieving measures
- ❖ Use individually titrated, regular analgesia so that the pain does not return
- ❖ Set realistic goals with the patient
- ❖ Analgesic drugs alone will not relieve all pain. Compassion, empathy, understanding, diversion and elevation of mood are essential complementary measures.
- ❖ If you are not successful in managing pain go back to the concept of total pain and ask, 'What have I missed'?

References

Farrar K (2001) Pain control. In: Gamlin R, Kinghorn S, eds. *Palliative Nursing: Bringing comfort and hope*. Baillière Tindall, Edinburgh

Frankl V (1959) *Man's Search for Meaning*. Simon and Schuster, New York

Gamlin R, Lovel T (2001) *Pain Explained: A guide for patients and carers*. Altman Publications, London

International Association for the Study of Pain (1986) Classification of chronic pain. Descriptions of chronic pain. Opioid requirements depend on previous analgesic needs syndromes and definitions of pain terms. *Pain* S3:1–226

McCaffery M (1972) *Nursing Management of the Patient in Pain*. JB Lippincott, Philadelphia

Melzack R, Wall PD (1982) *The Challenge of Pain*. Penguin, Harmondsworth

Mount BM (2003) Existential suffering and the determinants of healing. *Eur J Palliative Care* **10**(2)L: 40–2

Porta-Sales J, Gomez-Batiste X, Tuca-Rodriguez A, Madrid-Juan F, Espinosa-Rojas J, Trelis Navaro J (2003) Analgesic ladder — or lift? *Eur J Palliative Care* **10**(3): 105–9

Regnard CFB, Tempest S (1998) *A Guide to Symptom Relief in Advanced Cancer*. 4th edn. Haigh and Hochland, Manchester

Saunders CM (1967) *The Management of Terminal Illness*. Hospital Medicine Publications, London

Twycross R, Lack S (1984) *Symptom Control in Advanced Cancer*. Pitman Books, London

Twycross R, Wilcock A, Charlesworth S, Dickman A (2002) PCF2 *Palliative Care Formulary*. Radcliffe Medical Press, Oxford

World Health Organization (1986) *Cancer Pain Relief*. WHO, Geneva

World Health Organization (1996) *Cancer Pain Relief with a Guide to Opioid Availability*. WHO, Geneva

Useful websites

The American Pain Association
http://www.painfoundation.org/

StopPain.Org
http://www.stoppain.org

Chapter links to the NMC's *Code of Professional Conduct* (2002)

2. Respect the patient or client as an individual
    2.1 Partnership in care

2.2 Promote and respect dignity

3. Obtain consent before you give any treatment or care
   3.1 The right to information
   3.2 Respect for autonomy
   3.3 Presumption of competence
   3.11 The safe use of complimentary therapies

4. Cooperate with others in the team
   4.3 Communicate your skill, knowledge and expertise
   4.4 Ensure accurate record keeping

6. Maintain your professional knowledge and competence
   6.1 Participate in regular learning activities.

Chapter 5

Managing symptoms other than pain

I felt sick, I got a tablet, I couldn't breathe, I got another tablet. Now I can't go to the toilet. I watched the doctor write out another prescription. I hoped it would help but I was running out of faith. Along came Dawn. She asked me about everything and everything is now getting better.

Life threatening, progressing disease is a creeping crisis that invades patients, partners and carers alike. Although some will grow from the experience, it remains a distressing experience for all (Regnard and Tempest, 1998)

This chapter will consider the frequency of common symptoms in advanced illness and outline their management. Many excellent texts are available that discuss the detailed management of all common symptoms, for example, Regnard and Tempest (1998), Twycross, (1997), and Kaye, (1996).

Roper, Logan and Tierney (1980) said that the goal of nursing is to help patients to solve, alleviate or cope with problems they encounter. With all aspects of palliative care, and notably pain and symptom management, we may be able to solve problems but we have to live with the fact that we may not. Because of recent pharmacological and non-pharmacological developments we can almost always alleviate problems. We must never omit to help patients cope with their problems.

General principles of symptom management

⌘ Involve all appropriate members of the team.
⌘ Meticulous assessment: consider physical, psychological, spiritual and social factors.
⌘ Identify the patients concerns before the biochemical mechanisms.
⌘ Ask, 'what can I do to help?' and, 'What can my colleagues do to help?'
⌘ Listen attentively.
⌘ Show empathy.
⌘ Explain possible causes and treatment options.
⌘ Be vigilant for new symptoms and new causes for existing symptoms.
⌘ Review.

Hill (2000) provides a step by step approach to managing all symptoms:

1. List all the patient's symptoms.
2. Prioritise according to the patient's agenda.
3. List all possible causes of each symptom.
4. Establish probable diagnoses with full history, examination and investigations.
5. Establish patient's understanding of the problem.
6. Discuss possible cause(s) with the patient. Provide information.
7. Decide on appropriate treatment. Consider medical and non-medical interventions.
8. Individualise the treatment plan.
9. Set realistic goals and maintain hope.
10. Assess the response.
11. Review, review, review.

Frequency of common symptoms

Table 5.1 illustrates the frequency of common symptoms in advanced illness (collated by Atkinson and Virdee, 2001).

Table 5.1: Frequency of common symptoms in advanced illness		
Symptom	**Patients with cancer. % with symptom in last year of life**	**Patients with pro-gressive non-malignant disease. % with symptom last year of life**
Pain	84	67
Breathlessness	47	49
Vomiting or nausea	51	27
Sleeplessness	51	36
Confusion	33	38
Depression	38	36
Anorexia	71	38
Constipation	47	32
Pressure sores	28	14
Loss of bladder control	37	33
Loss of bowel control	25	22
Unpleasant smell	19	32

Symptoms are, all too often, managed in isolation rather than understanding that patients frequently have multiple symptoms with multiple causes.

Case study: Bill

Bill was a seventy-year-old man with cancer of the prostate. After a couple of days in hospital his pain was well controlled with a combination of morphine and diclofenac. Bill complained of nausea when talking to one nurse. He was given metoclopramide, an anti-emetic. Later that day he told another nurse he had abdominal pain. A different doctor prescribed Maalox, an antacid. He was discharged home a few days later and visited by his community nursing auxiliary. Bill told her he was having some problem going to the toilet. The nurse told the doctor who prescribed an antibiotic for a urinary tract infection.

The next day, Sally, the community staff-nurse went to see Bill. He appeared very unwell and perhaps depressed. Sally spent forty-five minutes with him assessing his pain and all his symptoms. She reported back to the GP and suggested a joint visit. The conclusions of the joint visit were:

- Bill's nausea was due to the morphine he began taking a few days ago. He was given haloperidol for this with excellent effect.
- The abdominal pain was due to the Diclofenac. His GP prescribed Lansoprazole that eased his pain two days later. Sally discussed Bill's eating habits and explained the importance of taking Diclofenac with meals.

When Sally asked him about, 'going to the toilet', Bill was a little embarrassed. He said, 'It's not my waterworks, it's the other'. Sally asked him how often he was going to the toilet and if it was difficult. Bill said, 'It's the piles, you know, they are very painful and it's very hard to go'. The GP examined Bill's anus and rectum. He found multiple haemorrhoids and a rectum full of hard faeces. Sally planned to come back later to give Bill a softening enema. The GP prescribed a stool softener and stimulant to treat the constipation. He also prescribed some ointment to reduce the pain and swelling around Bill's haemorrhoids. The antibiotic for Bill's non-existent urinary tract infection was stopped immediately.

Lessons to be learned

⌘ Patients commonly experience multiple symptoms. Assessing one symptom at a time may result in an incomplete assessment.

⌘ Medications to treat one symptom frequently cause another. For example, opioids used to treat pain can cause constipation and nausea.
⌘ Embarrassment, on the part of the patient or professional, may mask symptoms.
⌘ Listen to the patient.
⌘ Review.

Sally continued to visit daily. Each day Bill's condition improved. On day five, a smiling Bill greeted her at the door. He had no pain, nausea or constipation. Sally agreed to visit every few days to monitor these symptoms and to look for the development of anything new.

The remainder of the chapter will discuss the management of common symptoms

Nausea and vomiting

Nausea is a very unpleasant feeling familiar to us all, whereas vomiting is the act of being sick. Patients with advanced illness say that nausea is much worse than vomiting.

Vomiting mechanism

Vomiting is controlled by the vomiting centre in the brain. It is activated by stimuli from:

- the chemoreceptor trigger zone (CTZ)
- the upper gastrointestinal tract and pharynx
- the vestibular apparatus.

Higher centres in the cerebral cortex triggered by sounds, smells, worries and associations, for example, when the chemotherapy appointment arrives.

Causes of vomiting

There is a single cause in two thirds of patients.

CTZ

❖ Drugs such as opioids, chemotherapy, tricyclic antidepressants.

❖ Biochemical reasons such as hypercalcaemia, raised urea, renal and hepatic failure.

Vestibular

❖ Tumour
❖ Opioids
❖ Inner ear disturbance

Cerebral cortex

❖ Anxiety
❖ Raised intracranial pressure
❖ Association and previous experience

Peripheral

❖ Radiotherapy
❖ Chemotherapy
❖ Gastrointestinal irritation by pressure, inflammation or obstruction

Principles of management

Selecting appropriate anti-emetic drugs is essential. Likewise, are the other measures listed below:

- ensure privacy
- identify and treat the cause if possible
- manage the environment: Reduce unpleasant smells. Careful sensitive explanation
- offer mouth washes and preferred fluids in small amounts
- facilities to wash hands and face
- empty and replace vomit bowl immediately after vomiting. A large bowl is much better than a small 'kidney dish'
- measuring fluid balance may be necessary in protracted vomiting
- optimise non-pharmacological measures
- review at least every twenty-four hours.

Always ask: What is the likely cause of nausea and vomiting in this particular patient?

Anti-emetic therapy

⌘ Anticipate the need and give well before emetogenic stimulus.
⌘ Use adequate and regular doses.
⌘ Use appropriate route(s).
⌘ Aim at the appropriate receptor(s).
⌘ Combine drugs if more than one cause exists but keep regime as simple as possible.

Features and management of nausea and vomiting by cause

1. Gastric stasis

Features
Patient feels full. Often only slightly nauseated before vomiting. Vomit may be large and patient feels better after vomiting.

Management
If possible discontinue contributory medication or reduce dose. A prokinetic drug will help, for example, metoclopramide.

2. Intestinal obstruction

Features
Uncomfortable abdominal distension, generally unwell, may have colic. Large volume vomit is common. NB: It may be possible to treat the obstruction surgically. A surgical opinion should be sought.

Management
If no colic is present, subcutaneous metoclopramide, and a faecal softener. If colic is present, subcutaneous cyclizine and hyoscine butylbromide together with a faecal softener.

3. Biochemical disturbance

Features
Gradual onset with constant symptoms such as fatigue, confusion, and weakness anorexia and constipation. Nausea is usually constant.

Management

If possible and appropriate, correct the biochemical disturbance. Subcutaneous haloperidol.

4. Drugs

Features

There may be little to find on examination. Careful observation will reveal the relationship between consumption of drug and nausea.

Anticholinergics, chlorpromazine and opioids can cause gastric stasis Treat with metoclopramide.

NSAIDs, ampicillin, erythromycin, iron supplements, some cytotoxics can cause gastric irritation. Treat with metoclopramide and proton pump inhibitors (PPI).

Opioids, anticonvulsants, trimethoprim, metronidazole, ketoconazole, cytotoxics, some anaesthetic agents affect the CTZ. Treat with haloperidol.

NB: some drugs not noted for causing nausea, may cause nausea in some patients. Listen to the patient and believe them.

5. Raised ICP

Features

Onset may be gradual or sudden. Sensation of nausea may fluctuate. Neurological features such as paralysis, aphasia, amnesia and depression

Management

Steroids help by reducing oedema around the tumour. Cyclizine. Consider the role for radiotherapy, surgery or a shunt.

Constipation

> *When I got up this morning I took two ex-lax in addition to my Prozac. I can't get off the toilet, but I feel good about it.*

Constipation is a very common problem in advanced disease especially in patients taking opioids or with neurological disease. It can mimic the signs of advanced disease. It is embarrassing for patients to discuss therefore tact and diplomacy is required. In advanced disease it does not usually respond to exercise, increased fluid and fibre intake. Laxatives are almost always required.

What is constipation?

Constipation must never be defined by frequency of bowel action alone. It has been described as infrequent or difficult defaecation caused by decreased intestinal motility or a decrease in the frequency of the passage of formed stool characterised by stools that are hard and difficult to pass.

Signs and symptoms of constipation, include:

- difficulty in passing stool
- generalised or colicky abdominal pain
- distended abdomen
- flatulence
- anorexia and nausea
- increased or absent bowel sounds
- confusion
- diarrhoea: This should always be investigated. It may be due to loose stools bypassing hard faeces in the rectum. Treating with agents which firm the stool will make matters considerably worse. A digital rectal examination is essential.

Common causes of constipation, include:

- direct effects of cancer
- obstruction
- neurological damage
- hypercalcaemia
- secondary effects of advanced illness
- poor dietary and fluid intake
- weakness and immobility
- poor/unfamiliar toilet arrangements
- confusion
- drugs: opioids, tricyclic antidepressants, ant-parkinsonian agents, phenothiazines, hyoscine, diuretics, anticonvulsants, iron anti-hypertensives
- hypothyroidism
- hypokalaemia
- diabetes
- diverticular disease
- haemorrhoids, anal fissures/stenosis
- rectocele
- colitis.

Assessment

- ⌘ Sensitivity and **privacy**.
- ⌘ Discuss associated symptoms.
- ⌘ Identify normal bowel patterns. Frequency: 'What is it like when you go to the toilet?'
- ⌘ Usual bowel habits and changes in habits.
- ⌘ Drug regimes (prescribed and over the counter).
- ⌘ Worries and concerns: Constipation can mimic advanced abdominal cancer.
- ⌘ Toilet facilities and 'after toilet' facilities: disposal and hand-washing
- ⌘ Digital rectal examination.
- ⌘ Abdominal X-ray.
- ⌘ **Remember**: Frequency of bowel action, alone, is **not** a reliable indicator of constipation.

Management of constipation

- ⌘ Prevention of constipation is easier than treatment and should be the management strategy.
- ⌘ Regular bowel chart. This may appear 'old fashioned'. It can provide useful information.
- ⌘ Attention to diet. Maximise fluid and fibre intake.
- ⌘ Increase mobility.
- ⌘ Treatment of correctable causes.
- ⌘ Laxatives.
- ⌘ Home planning: modification may help.
- ⌘ Mouth care.
- ⌘ Food, fluids and supplements.
- ⌘ Education: explain about need to take medication regularly.

Manual evacuation: This procedure is occasionally necessary. Some paraplegic patients develop a regime whereby their stools are kept reasonably firm and they require manual evacuation every two or three days, but it is an unpleasant and undignified procedure. Skilled nursing will minimize distress. Careful explanation is essential. Some hospices carry out this procedure with sedation in very ill patients. The patient is given intravenous midazolam which has a sedative and amnesic action.

Laxatives

These should be given prophylactically. They usually have a softening, lubricant, stimulant or combined action. As with opioids dose titration is important. Some patients prefer laxatives that they have become accustomed to and this can aid compliance. Patients and carers need education to understand the principles of preventing constipation.

Most laxatives are well tolerated. Patients may be alarmed if they have red-urine after taking Danthron. It may also cause peri-anal skin irritation. Lactulose is safe and popular. Its sweet taste can be unpleasant for some and it may cause a feeling of fullness or cause colic. If constipation is caused by opioids, lactulose and senna appear to be equally effective but senna may be too 'severe' for some, causing griping abdominal pain.

Rectal preparations

Suppositories and enemas are sometimes required if other methods are ineffective. They should be avoided if at all possible. Careful explanation is needed so that patients know when to retain rectal preparations. The patients must be within easy access of toilet facilities. If they are weak help must be available.

Breathlessness

This can be a terrifying symptom with patients fearing death is near. Approximately one third of cancer patients and 70% of lung cancer patients will experience breathlessness. It is common in patients with chronic obstructive pulmonary disease (COPD) and cardiac failure. Patients may experience a sensation of suffocation, poor concentration, loss of appetite, loss of memory, profuse sweating and a feeling of isolation.

Common causes, include:

- primary tumour occluding an airway
- metastatic spread
- lymphatic occlusion
- COPD
- asthma
- pleural effusion
- pulmonary embolus
- anaemia
- pneumothorax
- chest infection
- cardiac failure

- renal failure leading to generalised oedema
- fear and anxiety
- superior vena-cava obstruction.

Management

Begin with a detailed assessment of breathlessness and factors which make it worse or better. Discuss and explain the meaning of breathlessness and its place in the illness. Patients often regard breathlessness as an inevitable consequence of lung cancer. Provide advice and support on methods of managing breathlessness for the patients and their family. A specialist nurse or physiotherapist can teach breathing retraining, relaxation and distraction while all nurses can help with goal setting to learn helpful techniques and integrate them into daily life. Early recognition of problems that may need drug treatment is important and general advice on maintaining health will optimise care

First consider simple but effective measures. Change the patients position. They may prefer to sit upright in a bed or chair supported by pillows. Circulating air reduces the subjective feeling of breathlessness. Open a window and provide a fan. Reduce overcrowding from staff and visitors to provide a calm atmosphere. Touch may relieve anxiety and relaxation exercises may help further. Plan the patient's day to conserve energy. Simple breathing exercises will help. Encourage the patient to breathe **out** slowly. It is frightening to be told to breathe slowly if you are fighting for breath. Involve the entire team where appropriate. A home assessment will reveal where additional equipment, nursing and social care will help. A specialist nurse, doctor or psychologist may help if anxiety and panic attacks are troublesome. Cognitive behavioural therapy can help in severe panic attacks.

Medication

- ⌘ Benzodiazepines such as diazepam, lorazepam and midazolam can bring symptomatic relief.
- ⌘ Small doses of oral morphine can help reduce the sensation of breathlessness. Morphine acts centrally to diminish the ventilatory drive stimulated by hypercapnia, hypoxia, and exercise.
- ⌘ Nebulised opioids act through a central as opposed to a local pulmonary mechanism. This is a relatively inefficient way of administering morphine.
- ⌘ Steroids will reduce swelling around the tumour.

Oxygen has been shown to improve exercise tolerance and prolong life in patients with COPD who are severely hypoxic. This may be due to the placebo effect but a cooling flow of oxygen against the face or through the nose may reduce breathlessness. Some patients keep an oxygen supply at the top and bottom of their stairs at home. Unfortunately, patients may become psychologically dependent on oxygen to such an extent that they are unable to go anywhere without it (Bredin *et al*, 1999)

For further information about nursing interventions to manage breathlessness see Bredin *et al* (1999).

Weakness and fatigue

Weakness and fatigue are common debilitating symptoms in advanced illness. The presence of other symptoms such as pain and nausea exacerbate weakness and fatigue and adversely affect patients' quality of life.

Possible causes of generalised weakness and fatigue, include:

- anaemia
- drugs
- sepsis
- metabolic imbalance
- cardiac, respiratory and renal failure
- lack of sleep and rest
- exhaustion due to the sheer weight of coping with the illness
- poor nutritional intake
- dehydration
- depression
- stress
- over activity.

Possible causes of localised weakness, include:

- localised trauma
- nerve damage
- spinal cord compression
- brain metastases
- neuropathy due to drug therapy.

Management of weakness and fatigue

- ⌘ Meticulous assessment.
- ⌘ Team approach, particularly physiotherapist and occupational therapist.
- ⌘ Treat reversible causes such as anaemia and electrolyte imbalance.
- ⌘ Enhance food and fluid intake.
- ⌘ Review medications.
- ⌘ Gentle exercise can enhance well-being.
- ⌘ Careful planning of the patient's environment and day.
- ⌘ Plan rest periods throughout day and enhance sleep.
- ⌘ Use aids to reduce energy expenditure. A wheelchair allows patients to 'scull' around home/ward and reduce energy expenditure.
- ⌘ Set realistic goals.
- ⌘ Steroids may provide short- or long-term benefit.

Anxiety and depression

There is a common misconception that anxiety and depression are inevitable consequences of advanced illness. Anxiety and depression do not always occur together but they are discussed together here.

Common causes of anxiety and depression, include:

- pre-existing mental health problems
- marital or relationship problems such as divorce and separation
- financial worries
- fear of illness, pain, loss, needles, chemotherapy, death, etc.
- lack of support from family and professionals
- drugs with an adrenaline-like action, such as salbutamol.

Assessment

- ~ *Can you tell me how you are feeling?*
- ~ *Do you know why you feel this way?*
- ~ *Do you have specific worries or concerns?*
- ~ *What do you think is going to happen to you?*
- ~ *How are you sleeping?*
- ~ *What do you think has caused you to feel this way?*
- ~ *Do you always feel so low or does it come and go?*
- ~ *How long have you felt like this?*

~ *Do you find you have lost interest in things around you?*
~ *Do you have any feelings of guilt? If so: Can you tell me about them?*
~ *What brought these feelings on?*

If a patient says or hints that they are feeling suicidal it must be taken seriously. They may have a treatable depression. They may actually have considered taking their own life. Clearly you must pass on your findings to a colleague, but remain supportive of the patient. You may ask:

~ *Have you actually thought about taking your own life?* If the answer is yes, carefully explore how the patient has considered taking their life. This will not encourage them to commit suicide.
~ *Does anyone else know you feel this way?*
~ *What might we do to help you feel better?*

Drug treatment

Anxiety may be managed using small doses of Benzodiazepines such as diazepam, midazolam or lorazepam. Beta-blockers such as propanolol can reduce the subjective feeling of anxiety by blocking the action of adrenaline, but they rarely help in patients with advanced illness.

Depression is commonly treated with selective serotonin reuptake inhibitors (SSRIs) such as fluoxetine (Prozac). Older antidepressant drugs, for example, tricyclic antidepressants such as amitriptyline can be of benefit. All antidepressants have side-effects. The gains must always be weighed against the possible benefits. Perceived prognosis is sometimes used as a reason for not prescribing antidepressant medications because they are not effective immediately. Judging prognosis is notoriously difficult; therefore they should not be withheld without meticulous assessment and planning involving the patient.

Non-drug measures

✺ Drugs offer symptomatic relief in the management of anxiety and depression. Some causes can be addressed and relieved. The continued presence of staff who will 'stay with' the patient through difficult times offers continued hope.
✺ Acknowledge the anxiety and provide someone to talk to, someone who will listen, someone who will give time.
✺ Discuss the reasons for anxiety and depression.

⌘ Simple jargon-free advice. It can be enormously helpful to know that a new pain is a muscle strain and not cancer which has spread.
⌘ Distraction: something to do.
⌘ Rest and sleep.
⌘ The support and advice of a community psychiatric nurse, GP, psychologist or psychiatrist.
⌘ Counselling.
⌘ Psychotherapy.
⌘ Cognitive behavioural therapy (CBT).

References

Atkinson J, Virdee A (2001) Promoting comfort for patients with symptoms other than pain. In Kinghorn S, Gamlin R, eds. *Palliative Nursing: Bringing comfort and hope*. Baillière Tindall, Edinburgh

Bredin M, Corner J, Krishnasamy M, Plant H, Bailey C, A'Hern R (1999) Multicentre randomised controlled trial of nursing intervention for breathlessness in patients with lung cancer. *Br Med J* **318**: 901–4. (RCT-119)

Hill S (2000) Symptom control. In: Cooper, ed. *Stepping into Palliative Care. A handbook for community professionals*. Radcliffe Medical Press, Oxford

Kaye P (1996) *A–Z Pocket Book of Symptoms*. EPL publications, Northampton

Regnard C, Tempest S (1998) *A Guide to Symptom Relief in Advanced Disease*. 4th edn. Hochland and Hochland, Cheshire

Roper N, Logan W, Tierney A (1980) *The Elements of Nursing*. Churchill Livingstone, Edinburgh

Twycross R (1997) *Symptom Management in Advanced Disease*. 2nd edn. Radcliffe Medical Press, Oxford

Useful websites

Managing constipation in advanced illness

http://www.albertapalliative.net/APN/PCHB/06_Constipation.html
http://www.painconsult.com/Pcc4.htm

Dyspnoea

http://www.in-touch.org.uk/Dyspnoea%20Case%20History%20Master.htm
http://www.vtsm.co.uk/data/clinical/decisions/guidelines_palliative_care.htm#Dyspnoea

Nausea and vomiting

http://www.jr2.ox.ac.uk/bandolier/booth/booths/pall.html
http://bmj.com/cgi/content/full/315/7116/1148
http://www.sea-band.com/The%20Sea%20Band/health.htm

Lymphoedema

http://www.lymphoedema.org/
http://www.cclf.co.uk/
http://www.cancerbacup.org.uk/info/lymphedema.htm

Depression

http://www.psychiatry.ox.ac.uk/cebmh/elmh/depression/index.html
http://www.psychiatry.ox.ac.uk/cebmh/elmh/depression/bibliography/index.html
http://cebmh.warne.ox.ac.uk/cebmh/whoguidemhpcuk/leaflets/07-1.html

Bowel obstruction

http://hospice.xtn.net//obstruct/

Chapter links to the NMC *Code of Professional Conduct* (2002)

2. Respect the patient or client as an individual
    2.1 Partnership in care
    2.2 Promote and respect dignity

3. Obtain consent before you give any treatment or care
    3.1 The right to information
    3.2 Respect for autonomy
    3.3 Presumption of competence
    3.11 The safe use of complimentary therapies

4. Cooperate with others in the team
    4.3 Communicate your skill, knowledge and expertise
    4.4 Ensure accurate record keeping

6. Maintain your professional knowledge and competence
    6.1 Participate in regular learning activities

Chapter 6

Essential comfort measures

Rosie was one of those nurses that always had a smile on her face... on one occasion she and a friend came to visit the ward after work and stopped by my bed just to see how I was getting on. I was okay that evening, the pain had gone, so they asked if they could get me something to eat. 'What do you fancy?' Rosie asked. 'A real Italian pizza with extra anchovies and pepperoni' I said. Sure enough, in about half an hour they returned smiling and shared with me the best pizza I had ever eaten.

Caring for the patient's body and immediate surroundings is probably the most common area of activity in any nurse's daily life. It is also the area that is most taken for granted in all healthcare practice (Lawler, 1991). A perceived neglect of the skills necessary in newly qualified nurses over the last ten years to care for the patients most essential needs was one of the major factors behind the Government's drive for better prepared nurses for practice. The nursing profession has had to look closely at its education curriculums for pre-registration nurses and to respond accordingly to remedy this situation (UKCC, 2001). The responsibility for such care is a shared one between qualified working nurses who provide the role models for good practice, and the educators who can supply the evidence base.

The *NHS Plan* (2000) reinforced to the nursing profession the importance of getting the essentials of care right and of improving the patient's experience. As a direct result of this document the *Essence of Care* (DoH, 2001) was launched to help practitioners take a much more patient focused and structured approach. This has now been developed into the *Essence of Care* (DoH, 2003) which attempts to set a range of benchmarks for standards in essential care and a toolkit for clinical areas to use to evaluate these standards.

These are important documents as they move back to centre stage this area of care which has often been referred to as basic care, implying that it involves unskilled tasks of low importance. Nothing could be further from the truth and this unfortunate attitude is demonstrated when the practice of keeping the patient's body clean and dry and the surrounding environment conducive to dignity and privacy is carried out as a routine and functional chore. The ever increasing numbers of healthcare assistants in all caring environments, whose job it is to carry out many of these activities, has in some ways indirectly contributed to the perception of such care as an unskilled activity and the techniques involved were, and probably still are, based more on tradition than valid research.

This chapter is intended to provide the nurse with a simple bulleted list of what will be referred to as essential comfort measures. It is not intended to be prescriptive, or to offer any particular framework or philosophical model, but simply to emphasise the vital importance of such care to the overall well being of our patients and those around the bedside. Such care has been described as sacred work, in which the carer enters into the intimate space of the patient and touches parts of the body that are usually private (Wolf, 1989). This is a highly privileged position that demands respect, a high degree of skill and sensitivity to individual need that is so essential when caring for the dying patient.

❖ *Privacy and dignity:* Consider such elements as the protection of modesty, the availability of some personal space for the patient, and respect for personal beliefs and identity (DoH, 2003).

❖ *Hair care:* Establish how often the patient likes their hair washed and conditioned and use the patient's own shampoo and conditioner where possible. Combs and brushes should be kept clean, and the hair blow dried preferably. Always make sure that the patient's hair is parted on the correct side and the trimming of beards and moustaches is done in accordance with the style that the patient is used to. Don't forget that excess hair protruding from the nose and ear may also need trimming, particularly with men. Use dry shampoo where appropriate.

❖ *Eyes:* Make sure that spectacles and/or contact lenses are clean — these often get overlooked — and use artificial tears to moisten the eyes where appropriate. Observe for signs of infection, such as redness around the eye or excessive discharge.

❖ *Mouth care:* Clean the teeth with the patient's preferred toothpaste, and/or dentures. Offer proprietary mouthwashes. Where the patient is immobile conduct an assessment of the mouth daily, and use Vaseline to moisten the lips or a lip salve stick if the patient prefers.

❖ *Ear care:* Use cleansing cotton buds gently around the visible area of the ear taking great care not to put the cotton buds too far inside the aural canal. Observe for ear wax build up and use wax softener where needed. If the patient's ears need syringing then seek the advice of the person in charge who will make arrangements for this procedure to be performed.

❖ ***Nose care:*** Clean with cotton buds daily and have soft tissues or hankies available.

❖ ***Nail care:*** Regular cleaning and trimming and shaping for both men and women will keep nails looking good. Observe for infections, ie. athletes foot, cuticle care, dry split skin, and refer to a chiropodist if there are visible malformations, such as corns or bunions.

❖ ***Massage:*** One of the simplest and most therapeutic forms of touch a nurse can ever use with a patient. It is not necessary to attend a course or be formally qualified to use gentle massage on the hands and feet as long as simple safety precautions are observed. Establish that this is acceptable to the patient, some cultures may find it offensive and there may be gender issues. Talk to the patient where possible to establish that there are no open cuts, or abrasions, and no arthritic or swollen joints. If there are any other lesions or tumours visible, then massage is clearly contraindicated. Find out what is available and what the patient prefers in terms of hand creams, or perhaps aromatherapy oils.

❖ ***Odours:*** Strong smells around a bedside are both embarrassing for the patient and family and avoidable in most cases. Be aware that the spray deodorisers that are readily available in most clinical areas are not suitable, as they can cause allergic sneezing reactions and increase restlessness in an unconscious patient. Simple aromatherapy oils are very effective and cheap and easy to obtain. Use relevant charcoal infused dressings to absorb odours from wounds. Fungating wounds sometimes need to be treated with metronidazole.

❖ ***Bodily hygiene:*** Whilst the patient is capable, regular baths or showers as suits the patients' choice. Use a jacuzzi if available. If the patient is close to death then full bed baths are intrusive and inappropriate at such a sensitive time, so establish when and when not to.

❖ ***Wound care:*** Make sure that all dressings are secure and there is a regular assessment of wound condition. If the patient is in pain, consider appropriate analgesia before dressing times.

❖ ***Environmental issues:*** Maximise natural lighting around the patient's bedside where possible. It is well known that a person's visual acuity deteriorates as they approach death, therefore the temptation to dim the lights should be avoided. Try to avoid unnecessary clutter on and around the bed and make sure that there is good ventilation and warmth. Use natural flowers checking that the patient has no known allergies or dry flowers instead. Look also at neighbouring patients: are they chatty or are they dying? Do they have lots of visitors?

❖ *Creative crafts:* Diversional therapy such as card making, knitting, painting, jigsaw puzzles and games can be very helpful to the patient.

❖ *Diet/nutrition:* The key things to remember are small, well-presented meals, high in calories to boost energy. Assessment of nutritional likes and dislikes should be made and meals should be modified to suit the patient's wishes with liberal interpretations of diabetic needs. If feeding is needed, time should be allowed for this important and often neglected function.

❖ *Belongings:* Making a patient's bed space personal to them is psychologically very important in any caring environment away from the home. Encourage the use of photos, personal clothes and jewellery.

❖ *Entertainment:* Newspapers, magazines, books, TV with remote control, CDs and radios, walkmans, headphones and, of course, plenty of batteries. Consider the use of games consoles if available, not only with young people, but adults can get a lot of enjoyment from them.

❖ *Visits:* Find out from the patient who is important in their life and do not always assume that it is immediate family. Be aware that the patient may tire easily with too many people around and be their advocate when necessary to limit time spent at the bedside. Find out what the visiting policy is and remember issues such as parking, refreshments, and chairs around the bed. Consider open visiting if the family travel a long distance. The key element is to remain discreetly in the background, but available.

❖ *Pets:* There is an increasing body of evidence that visiting pets around the bedside in clinical areas is good for the patient as it increases self-esteem, helps the patient maintain what for them could be a very important relationship with their pet and reinforces a sense of normality. Find out beforehand; who will bring the animal and keep control of it, if there are any behavioural issues to consider, and if the pet is house trained. Also, establish if any of the nearby patients are allergic to the animal itself. Once these simple precautions are observed most areas are now happy to accommodate short visits and the other patients often enjoy observing the pet. Consider contacting the local 'Pets as Therapy' representative, who can arrange for a visitor to bring in their pets. This is a national charity who carefully screen all animals prior to allowing them to visit a clinical area.

❖ ***Make up:*** Looking and feeling normal is important for all of us and cosmetics, perfume, deodorant, after shave all form part of this. Find out what the patient prefers and be prepared to help them apply the make up if necessary.

❖ ***Sleep and rest:*** Make sure that there are quiet periods for the patient, reduce intrusive noise, ie. TV, radio, medication trolleys. Consider alternatives to sleep inducing agents, ie. Horlicks, Ovaltine, small amounts of alcohol and ear plugs.

❖ ***Mobility:*** Passive exercises are part of the nursing role, but consider also assessment by a physiotherapist and an occupational therapist where necessary. Shoes should be well fitting, any aids for walking readily available and positioning of the patient in chair or bed is crucial to comfort.

❖ ***Bowel care:*** Awareness of opioids and other medication and their effect on the bowels. Consider intervention every third day if the bowels have not opened. Never forget issues of privacy and dignity.

❖ ***Elimination:*** If diuretics are prescribed establish the timing of this medication. If a catheter is *in situ* then check for infections, blockages and observe the colour and consistency of the urine. If the patient has specifically requested that a catheter not be inserted when they become incapable this should be respected.

❖ ***Futile medications:*** When the patient is close to death a regular review of the total regime is crucial. The whole care team should ask themselves whether IV infusions, TPN feeding, and the use of subcutaneous fluids are useful and appropriate. The decision to withdraw such treatment is ethically, morally and legally appropriate if the team agrees that it is in the patient's best interest. The family's views should be listened too and acknowledged, but are secondary in this instance.

❖ **Routine observations:** It is not necessary to record temperature, pulse respirations or blood pressure on a patient who is clearly dying, except where instructed for clear medical reasons, for example, when a procedure such as a blood transfusion is in progress.

References

Department of Health (2001) *Essence of Care*. DoH, London

Department of Health (2003) *Essence of Care: Patient focused benchmarks for clinical governance*. DoH, London

Department of Health (2000) *The NHS Plan: A Plan for Investment, A Plan for Reform*. The Stationery Office, London.

Lawler J (1991) *Behind the Screen: Nursing, somology and the problem of the body*. Churchill Livingstone, Melbourne.

United Kingdom Central Council for Nursing, Midwifery and Health Visiting Post Commission Development Group (2001) *Fitness for Practice and Purpose*. UKCC, London

Wolf ZR (1989) Uncovering the hidden work of nursing. *Nurs Health Care* **10**(8): 462–7

Useful websites

Essence of Care Programme

http://www.doh.gov.uk/essenceofcare

Pets as Therapy

http://www.petsastherapy.org

Chapter links to the NMC's *Code of Professional Conduct* (2002)

2. Respect the patient or client as an individual
   2.1 Partnership in care
   2.2 Promote and respect dignity

6. Maintain your professional knowledge and competence
   6.5 Deliver care based on evidence, research and best practice

Chapter 7

Caring for the bereaved

We had been together for over forty years, Tom and I. I loved him, at times I hated him. He was my life, my love, my inspiration, my reason to be. Now he is dead. This is not how I planned it. My heart **screams** out with pain and every sentence begins with, 'if only'.

Throughout life we experience many losses and constant change. According to Littlewood (1992), a quarter of the world's population will be experiencing the death of someone close who has died in the last five years. Josef Stalin said, 'The death of one person is a tragedy, the death of a million is a statistic'. To all patients, and those who love them, loss is a tragedy. For staff who care for patients their death is never merely a statistic.

The nature of loss

Loss affects us in different ways depending on the type and frequency of the loss or change. Grief must be suffered if we are to adjust to our loss and carry on with life, although life will never be quite the same. We become used to responding quickly and efficiently to the problems of the dying, but dealing with loss is quite different. There are no quick fix answers. Nevertheless, there is much that can be done to support the bereaved.

When we think of loss in the context of palliative care we naturally think of death. If you think back over your own life you will be able to think of other losses. Moving house aged eleven results in the loss of a way of life and friends. Leaving home aged eighteen to start work, university or to marry results in enormous changes. Broken relationships as a result of divorce or separation, redundancy, infertility, illness and momentous world events all affect us to some extent.

Think back to some of the losses you have suffered during your life and make a list of some of the emotions that you experienced. It is likely that you felt some of the following:

- pain
- anger

- distress
- bewilderment
- relief
- guilt
- mistrust
- emptiness
- loneliness
- distress
- confusion.

Time softens some of the emotions but sometimes a memory, a smell or a song can bring them back into sharp focus. The process of coming to terms with loss takes a long time and the journey is scattered with pitfalls. As professionals, we must remember this and provide continued support.

Some comments made by the bereaved

~ *It's so lonely.*
~ *It hurts, a gut wrenching pain. Will it ever go away?*
~ *He was here, always here, now I have nothing but a hollow emptiness.*
~ *Why why why? I would do anything to bring her back.*
~ *If only...*
~ *I never told him I loved him.*
~ *Life has been hard, I just want to feel whole again.*

How can we help?

We have built up a picture of what loss is and how it affects people. It is helpful to consider how we may support the bereaved. Ask any professional what is difficult about caring for the dying and bereaved and many will respond, 'I don't know what to say'. We must remember that nothing will 'fix' the problem or make it all better. Often we resort to empty platitudes we have learned as we grew up, for example:

~ *He had a good innings.*
~ *At least he is not suffering any more.*
~ *At least he is not in pain.*
~ *You will find someone else.*
~ *I know how you feel.*
~ *You have still got the twins.*

~ *Time is a healer*
~ *You just have to get on with life.*
~ *Look on the bright side.*

These comments do not help apart from making us think that we have done something.

What can I say?

The bereaved feel even more lonely and isolated when they are ignored by family, friends and professionals. Meeting someone who is bereaved, for the first time, is difficult because we fear making it worse. This is very unlikely so we must try to find words of comfort. There are no magical answers, but the following may sometimes help:

~ *I don't know what to say.*
~ *I can only imagine how difficult this must be for you.*
~ *Would you like me to stay?*
~ *I am sorry for your loss.*
~ *Would you like to talk?*
~ *Is there anything I can do to help?*
~ *How are you?*
~ *How do you feel?*
~ *Do you have any questions?*

The course of grief is summed up so eloquently by Lewis (1961):

> *Grief is like a long valley, a winding valley where any bend may reveal a totally new landscape... sometimes the surprise is the opposite one: you are presented with exactly the same sort of landscape you thought you left behind miles ago.*

What else can I do?

Taking that first step is so important. Following up is equally important. Don't underestimate the value of making a cup of tea and sitting with the newly bereaved. You will feel that you have done something and the bereaved will appreciate the kindness. The bereaved value someone who will listen and stay with them through the pain.

What else can I do to support the bereaved?

❖ *By being there:* Don't attempt to offer any solutions, because there are none. In addition to practical help in the early stages do not underestimate the value of being there and listening. Your 'presence' can be invaluable.

❖ *By active listening in a non-judgmental way:* Allow people time to grieve in a way that suits them. There is no right or wrong way to grieve.

❖ *Be clear in your intentions:* If you make a conscious decision to stay and help the person, commit yourself to this decision.

❖ *Accept that you cannot make them better:* This is a different kind of helping. In order for people to grieve successfully they must experience the pain that goes with it.

❖ *Allow sadness:* Take their feelings and fears seriously and reinforce to them the normality of their experiences.

❖ *Expect anger:* This is a normal reaction and should not be taken personally. They may be angry with you, the doctors, god or even the person who has died.

❖ *Encourage them to talk of the deceased:* Ask about their life together and look at mementos and photographs. Allow them to tell their story as they see it.

❖ *Allow repetition:* This is very common and is known to be helpful. It helps the bereaved to make sense of what has happened.

❖ *Mention the deceased by name:* This helps to affirm your interest and encourages expression. 'I enjoyed caring for Bill and hearing him talk of his love for you'.

❖ *Appropriate physical contact:* Use touch in a caring sensitive way if you feel it is the right thing to do.

❖ *Tolerate silences:* People can do a lot of useful thinking in silent moments. Resist the urge to speak.

❖ **Develop hope:** Reassure them that difficult feelings are part of grief and that it is normal and self limiting.

❖ **Be familiar with your own feelings in this area:** You need to have thought through your own reactions to death and dying. In particular, with past events and scars.

Models of grief

Many models of grief exist. Their purpose is to help the reader to understand the nature and complexity of loss and to offer insights into helping the bereaved. They can be categorised as phase models, the medical model, grief work models and the grief bereavement biography model. For an excellent critical review of loss models see Anstey and Lewis (2001).

Perhaps the most useful loss model in palliative care is Worden's model (1991), which proposed four tasks of mourning the bereaved must attend to. These are:

1. Accept the reality of the loss.
2. Experience and work through the pain of grief.
3. Adjust to life without the deceased.
4. Emotionally relocate the deceased and move on with life.

Looking at these tasks and drawing on your personal experience one can sense the enormity of these tasks when someone loses a loved one. It may be useful to think about and list the sort of things that have helped you to cope. You may have thought of the following:

- practical help: child-care, shopping
- someone who will listen and not tell me what to do
- someone who will let me tell my story over and over again
- my faith
- crying
- quiet contemplation.

In addition, the following suggestions are presented to help you apply Worden's model (1991).

Worden's task	Ways of helping
Accept the reality of the loss	Talk to the bereaved
	Use clear explicit language: dead and death rather than gone or passed on
	Stay with the bereaved
	Speak of the dead
	Repeat the bad news
	Listen and explain
Experience and work through the pain of grief	Listen and help the bereaved tell their story
	Acknowledge the pain, anger and distress
Adjust to life without the deceased	Revisit the story
	Talk about the deceased
	Practical advice about work, life, money, relationships
	Revisit feelings
	Explore fears
Emotionally relocate the deceased and move on with life	Rituals, eg. services of remembrance
	Help the deceased to say goodbye and move on without forgetting the one who has died
	Talk about other relationships

Case study: Josh

To conclude this chapter you may like to consider Josh and think about how you could offer him help and support.

Josh is a fifty-year-old university lecturer. He was born in Hull and moved to Edinburgh when he was eleven. His grandmother died when Josh was twenty-one and his father died suddenly when he was thirty-two. A very close friend moved to America ten years ago. He separated from his wife and son eighteen months ago. His mother, with whom he has always been very close, is now frail and elderly. Josh is unremarkable yet he has suffered a number of major losses throughout his life. It is likely that he will also have experienced many other losses.

While in hospital for minor surgery you notice he is quiet and withdrawn. You ask how he is feeling and offer an opportunity to talk. He talks freely and openly about many things, including:

- his feelings about his dad and things left unsaid
- his marriage, his sense of failure and being judged by others
- his feelings towards his son he misses every day
- his fears about losing his mother in the coming years
- his uncertainty about his future and the possibility of finding love again.

After listening for a while you ask if it is possible for Josh to sum up how he feels at the moment. He talks eloquently of past pleasures and pains. 'Good friends jolly me along reassuring me that it will get better'. 'I have an overwhelming and all-consuming feeling of loneliness and missed opportunities as I struggle with each day'.

When you listen to Josh you may think he should not have left his wife or he should have spent more time with his mum. Like it or not, we are all judgmental to some extent. The judgments we make are influenced by our culture, upbringing, education and the team in which we work. Be aware of your judgments. Talk them through with a trusted colleague so that you can put them in perspective. We may not be totally at ease with, for example, homosexuality, infidelity or asylum seekers but we have to find a way to live with our judgments and provide care for the dying and bereaved.

Risk assessment of those facing bereavement

Student nurses are inevitably close to patients and families on a physical and emotional level. They are in a unique position to contribute to the assessment of bereavement risk. Carrying out bereavement risk assessment aims to reduce the long-term effects of unresolved grief and target scarce resources available to the bereaved. Melliar-Smith (2002) provides a detailed account of how to perform bereavement risk assessment together with a document developed by herself and her colleagues. Consider the following aspects surrounding the illness, death and relationships between the carer and the patient:

⌘ Length of time patient has been in your care.
⌘ Mode of death: sudden, peaceful or problematic.
⌘ Main carers understanding of illness and care.
⌘ Spiritual and religious issues.
⌘ Anticipatory grieving: Have the patient and carers discussed death and putting affairs in order.

⌘ Previous life events experienced by carers: other deaths, physical or mental illness or trauma, divorce, separation, financial problems, dependent children and other relatives, employment, family conflict
⌘ Carers health: physical and emotional.
⌘ Any other issues that may affect the carer's bereavement. Taking the above issues into consideration and your 'gut feeling', discuss your assessment of the patient's risk of a bereavement that could remain unresolved with your colleagues.

Anticipatory grief

It is essential to understand that grief does not begin when the patient dies and the survivors are alone. Lindemann (1994) described grief which occurs before the death in anticipation. The concept of anticipatory grief can be used to understand reactions leading up to death. At present there appears to be no convincing evidence that anticipatory grief work modifies the bereaved's response to loss. This should not deter all staff from acknowledging losses that have and continue to occur, including approaching death.

References

Anstey S, Lewis M (2001) Bereavement, grief and mourning. In: Kinghorn S, Gamlin R, eds. *Palliative Nursing: Bringing Comfort and Hope*. Baillière Tindall, Edinburgh

Lewis CS (1961) *A Grief Observed*. Faber & Faber, London

Lindemann E (1994) Symptomatology and the management of acute grief. *Am J Psychiatry* 101: 141–8

Littlewood J (1992) *Aspects of Grief: Bereavement in adult life*. Routledge, London

Melliar-Smith C (2002) The risk assessment of bereavement in a palliative care setting. *Int J Palliative Nurs* **8**(6): 281–7

Worden W (1991) *Grief Counselling and Grief Therapy*. Tavistock Routledge, London

Organisations and websites that offer support to the bereaved

Child Death Helpline
http://www.childdeathhelpline.org
telephone: 0800 282986;
address: The bereavement services dept
Great Ormond St Hospital

Great Ormond St, London, WC1N 3JH
Childhood Bereavement Network
http://www.ncb.org.uk
telephone: 0115 9118070
address: Huntingdon House
278–290 Huntingdon St,
Nottingham NG1 3LY

Cruse Bereavement Care
http://www.cruseberavement.org.uk
telephone: 0208 9399530
address: Cruse House
126 Sheen Rd
Richmond
Surrey
TW9 1UR

Compassionate Friends
http://www.tcf.org.uk
telephone 0117 9665202
address: 53 North St
Bristol
BS3 1EN

Samaritans
http://www.samaritans.org.uk
telephone: 01753 531011; local branches in telephone directory

Chapter links to the NMC's *Code of Professional Conduct* (2002)

2. Respect the patient or client as an individual
    2.1 Partnership in care
    2.2 Promote and respect dignity
    2.4 Help patient's gain access to information and support.

Chapter 8

Communicating with care and compassion

> I lay on my bed, terrified and isolated, watching and listening. I know
> I have cancer, the consultant told me two weeks ago. It was as if
> nothing had happened. Nurses dashed past with their busy masks.
> Doctors towered over me chanting their jargon. Had anyone any
> idea what I felt like? Did anybody care?

The doctor-patient relationship is founded on trust, it is nurtured by honesty and poisoned by deceit (Twycross, 1995).

All patient-professional relationships are similarly based on trust and skilled communication is at the very heart of palliative care. Without effective compassionate communication it is not possible to achieve trust, manage pain and symptoms, to comfort the bereaved or ease spiritual distress. Ensuring that all involved in the patient's care receive appropriate and timely information and support is enormously complex, requiring attention to detail and commitment. Students of health care spend much of their time in direct patient care. Consequently, opportunities to really make a positive contribution to care are always present. The words of Stephen Covey (1989), 'Seek first to understand, then to be understood', form a useful foundation for all communication — be it with patients, families or colleagues. Listen carefully, don't be in a hurry to find a simple solution to complex problems and take every opportunity to communicate effectively. Your patients and their families will never forget you.

Dunlop (Grove, 1999) suggests that we are literally the patient's servant. We must ask, he believes:

What is it that you feel you need? I am here as your textbook.
Open me at whatever page you feel you think might be helpful.

He goes on to discuss complex questions, such as when a patient expresses a wish to end their life. This question must be explored because it is usually related to depression, feeling a burden, or it may be because of pain or other symptoms. The patient deserves an exhaustive search for palliative alternatives, after which some change their minds about wanting to die. Our job is not to ignore a request but to discuss it.

For some it may seem daunting to address such fundamental questions about life and death. 'I am only a student', seems a perfectly reasonable excuse. In time you will be only a staff nurse, then only a sister. If you don't have the courage to face issues such as this we guarantee they will not become easier if you leave them until you are 'older and wiser'. Remember this: The patient chose you because they trusted you. Avoiding the question not only leaves the patient still searching but undermines the trust Twycross puts firmly at the centre of all we do. Please remember that dying people prefer to talk about life rather than death and dying. Most conversations with dying patients are not about death or dying but we must be ready to 'change gear' if and when necessary.

Listening and the value of silence

It seems a little odd to be discussing silence at the beginning of a chapter on communication. Silence is when nothing happens... or is it? Resist the urge to fill silences. The patient's mind will be far from empty; he will be searching for words to express complex and perhaps tragic feelings. Throughout life most of us get little opportunity to do this. We find it difficult to express our thoughts, feelings and needs when we are fit and well. When we are ill it is much more difficult. It is hard to find the right words and our thoughts become confused. When we are in this frame of mind, remember that the slightest interruption can break our train of thought and set us back a long way. Just as spaces are needed on a page to emphasise the words, so pauses and silences in a conversation are necessary to emphasise what is being said (Booth, 2000). Find a colleague who has these skills and observe carefully. Psychologists and psychiatric nurses tend to use silences as a basis for listening.

Listening is a complex and active process. In essence, it requires that we give our full and undivided attention to another person. Sitting down and making gentle eye contact send the powerful message: I am here for you. In the course of listening we use skills with which you will be familiar.

Listening and attending skills

Paraphrasing consists of putting the patients words into our own words, while reflecting indicates that we are trying to understand the patient's feelings. Summarising during and towards the end of a conversation allows us to piece together the patient's story and check that we have understood. At times, although this may sound harsh, we may need to challenge and

patient's behaviour. Aim for most of your questions to be open
ree-flowing conversation, but closed questions have their place
ng factual questions. Two simple questions to ask yourself about
versations with a patient are: 'Is this nurse or patient-centred'?
doing most of the talking?' If it is nurse-centred or you are doing
the talking, think about how you can redress the balance.
ful questions/statements prompts to develop your conversation:

> *Would you like to talk?*
> *Would you like to tell me what's on your mind?*
> *What is it really like to be you?*
> *~ What's troubling you?*
> *~ In the time that's left, what is important to you?*
> *~ Is there anything I can say/do to help?*
> *~ How do you feel now you have had a chance to speak to the
>   doctor?*
> *~ Have you any regrets?*
> *~ Is there anything you can do to put things right?*
> *~ What do you really enjoy?*
> *~ Tell me what it was like to be an engineer/manager/teacher?*

Sensitive listening, attending and questioning will have enormous benefits
for patients and staff. According to Jones (1999), patients can look without
a single word and convey the message, 'I know you know'. As Doyle
illustrates, patients work out a lot for themselves:

> *You don't normally spend two weeks in hospital having your whole
> body x-rayed and gallons of blood taken for tests if you have got
> flu, do you doctor?*

> *If a doctor gives it to you straight you're ok because they never do
> that if it's cancer. If it's the big C, doctors waffle.*

Does the patient know? Does the patient want to know?

Much pain can unwittingly be caused by staff and relatives who make
assumptions about what the patient knows and wants to know about their
illness. Patients often have a very good idea about what is wrong with
them. Consider Jim, a sixty-eight-year-old man who has smoked for almost
fifty years. As he chats with his doctor about his worsening chest condition
and the new terrifying symptom, haemoptysis, it is very unlikely that the

possibility of cancer has not crossed his mind. Finding out what
knows **and** wants to know is the key to dealing with this comple

A conversation between Jim and his GP:

Jim: *This has got me worried this time doctor.*
GP: *What's going through your mind this time Jim?*
Jim: *Well, you put 2 and 2 together don't you?*
GP: *Do you want to tell me what you come up with or is that a bit
       Jim?*
Jim: *It's far too scary!*
GP: *Are you ready for me to tell you what I have come up with?*
Jim: *Umm... yes doc, but no gory details, just lay it out on the line...*
GP: *You quite sure Jim?*
Jim: *Go for it as the kids say these days.*
GP: *This could be another chest infection or your bronchitis getting
       worse but I am more concerned today because of the blood... Sha
       I tell you what's on my mind?*
Jim: *Yes please, I have to know.*
GP: *Jim there is a strong possibility that you may have lung
       cancer... Is that a shock to you?*
Jim: *Yes and no... I have ignored the warnings on the packets but you
       always hope it you will get away with it... What's next doc?*

The GP then went on to discuss investigations. He offered to talk about
treatment options should the diagnosis be confirmed, but Jim declined.

What can we learn from this?

⌘   Serious illness is not always a complete shock but is almost always
     frightening.
⌘   Patients will tell you what they want to know if you allow them to.
⌘   Use simple language and go at the patient's pace.

For further information about breaking bad news see Buckman (1998) and
Buckman (1992).

Developing our conversations

We may need to ask direct questions about sensitive issues rather than waiting for the patient to ask us. If you find this difficult it may be because you do not want to distress the patient. Alternatively, it may be because you wish to avoid confronting your own pain and fear. Think carefully about this and find someone to talk to. When teaching we regularly encounter students who become upset. When talking with them they tell us about what has upset them. Often they tell of events in the distant past that they have not confronted. They may decide to discuss such issues with a GP, counsellor or psychologist. Acknowledging and telling the story can be sufficient to resolve what has happened. Others deal with traumatic events by 'filing them away' in the mind and using denial. This is one way of coping and sometimes an effective way, but, be aware that this could have a negative effect on your ability to help patients. If in doubt, seek some confidential advice.

Spending time with patients

In the past, nurses who spent time with patients were sometimes criticised and frequently felt guilty. Times have changed but old habits and customs change slowly. Nowadays, nursing is conducted at a rapid pace with high patient turnover and discharge pressures. We feel that something else is always more important and we must be seen to be doing.

A little time spent with a patient, listening and responding with care and compassion may have greater therapeutic value than any clinical procedure (Anstey, 1991). 'We haven't got time' is the perfect reason or excuse for not spending time with a patient. Even five minutes sitting on the bed may be all the patient wants if you are ready to listen and be prepared to answer questions honestly and simply. They don't want a one-sided conversation devoid of substance or, worse still, one which is patronising and full of platitudes (Doyle, 1999).

Caring and showing compassion will not be perceived by your patients as proportional to the time spent with them. You will be judged by the relationship that you develop and your ability to demonstrate respect, compassion, love and understanding.

Modern influences on communication: The *NHS Plan* and the *Cancer Plan*

In recent years much emphasis has been placed on national service frameworks. The *NHS Plan* and the *Cancer Plan* offer guidance about the communication needs of patients and their families.

> *The NHS Plan will introduce new joint training across professions in communication skills. By 2002 it will be a precondition of qualification to deliver patient care in the NHS that staff are able to demonstrate competence in communication with patients. For cancer we will give additional training in communication skills and psychological support.*

Students receive communication skills training but, frequently, find difficulties in relating theory to practice. Our students will continue to be taught more about the chemistry of the body than the alchemy of relationships (Doyle, 1999).

Sadly, patients report being given bad news and other information in a deeply insensitive way, being left in the dark about their condition and being badly informed about their treatment and care. Surveys of cancer patients have shown that they give a high priority to:

- being treated with humanity, with dignity and respect
- good communication with health professionals
- being given clear information about their condition
- receiving psychological support when they need it.

Further developing communication skills

This is a lifelong process. We learn our skills by watching and listening to others.

⌘ Identify your own style. Listen carefully to yourself and ask trusted colleagues to give you honest feedback.
⌘ Listen attentively to others: reflect carefully on their style, accept their strengths and reject their weaknesses. Note useful phrases and gestures. Don't attempt to learn a script but adapt the style of colleagues.
⌘ Practice, practice, practice: role play with fellow students, colleagues and lecturers. Ask for feedback. Tape your practice and review.

Giving information

Patients need information: information that is intelligible, that they can make sense of. Think back to the days before you were a student. Would you understand, for example, bronchoscopy, biopsy, oncology and prognosis? In our quest for providing information there is a danger that we give too much. Look at the amount of cancer information that is available, such as leaflets, booklets, videos and tapes. Some is excellent but some is poorly constructed and presented. If you choose to give written information, read it carefully so that you know the contents. If you are working on a ward where you feel the written information could be improved, bring it to the attention of the senior staff. Healthcare staff often criticise patients for using information found on the Internet. Criticism is futile and unhelpful. If a patient or relatives mentions Internet information, ask to see it and help them to make sense of it. A qualified colleague may be able to give an honest appraisal of its value.

Principles of giving information

- ⌘ Where possible, plan ahead. Think about what you will say.
- ⌘ Give information in small chunks.
- ⌘ **Stop** and gauge reaction.
- ⌘ Invite questions.
- ⌘ Clarify.
- ⌘ Give a little more information.
- ⌘ **Stop** and gauge reaction.
- ⌘ Invite questions.
- ⌘ Summarise.
- ⌘ Invite questions.
- ⌘ Final check.

As a final check we commonly ask, 'Do you understand?' Most patients will say 'yes'. Try saying something like, 'We have talked about a lot of things, can I just check I have explained clearly. Please can you tell me what you understand from what I have said'. You may be surprised to hear that your clear message has not been received and understood but you have an opportunity to explain again.

We should expect patients to retain only a small proportion of what we tell them so it is essential to go back later that day or soon after. It is likely that they may have thought of some questions to ask you.

Case study: Steven

Steven was admitted to a surgical ward after having had investigations for a hoarse voice. The next day he was to have a laryngectomy and would be nursed in intensive care for a few days.

At the time I was a clinical teacher running the intensive care course. On the day before Steven's surgery I took a student nurse with me to complete a pre-operative visit.

We greeted Steven, introduced ourselves and I explained the purpose of our visit: To tell Steven what would happen to him when he came to the intensive care unit.

'Can I stop you there son', Steven said with a hint of anger in his voice and in his eyes. 'I have been seen by the house officer, the senior house officer, the registrar, the consultant. I have been seen by the theatre nurse, the anaesthetic nurse and now you two. All of them have told me what they are going to do to me, how it won't hurt it will just be uncomfortable and oh, by the way, you won't be able to talk but you can just write down what you want.'

'No-one has told me how I am going to cope with all this. Oh and by the way, I can't write even though I run a business. Most of their sentences finished with OK? All right? No it isn't ok, it's bloody terrifying. You lot just haven't a bloody clue.'

Dealing with difficult questions: sometimes sharing a question is more important than answering it.

In the Harry Potter story, *The Philosopher's Stone*, Dumbledore the Headmaster says:

> *The truth is a beautiful and a terrible thing and should therefore be treated with great caution. However I shall answer your questions unless I have a good reason not to, in which case, I beg you to forgive me. I shall not of course tell a lie.*

> Rowling, 1997

Patients do ask direct questions but be alert for difficult questions hidden behind a mask. Patients who mask their difficult questions are generally too frightened to ask them outright. Unfortunately, they are easy to miss.

Some examples of openly difficult question, include:

~ *How long have I got?*
~ *Does this mean the cancer has come back?*
~ *What will it be like?*
~ *You won't let me die in pain will you?*
~ *Have I got cancer?*
~ *Am I going to die?*
~ *Will you put me out of my misery?*

Some examples of 'masked' difficult questions, include:

~ *I seem to be losing so much weight, I wonder what that can be?*
~ *Do you get many patients in here with this?*
~ *My uncle had something like this and well he...*
~ *These tablets don't seem to be making any difference do they?*
~ *I wonder how John will cope in the future?*

All these questions are difficult either because we do not know the answer or the answer will cause pain and distress. A difficult question should be the stimulus for a dialogue and not merely something that requires a simple answer.

When a patient asks us a difficult question they have usually thought long and hard and chosen someone that they can trust. They expect an honest response demonstrating that we understand and wish to help. Often we will not know the full answer including all the clinical details. It is not a failing to admit this. If we try to bluff our way out we will be discovered and we will destroy the trust.

Responding to the question: How long have I got?

Check out the meaning of the question. 'How long have I got?' may mean before I die or before I go to X-ray. A possible response would be: 'When you say, How long have I got? Could I ask what you mean by that?'

If the patient says, 'before I die' this requires careful handling. You could go on and say, 'I am wondering why you ask me that'. The patient may describe his thoughts feelings and fears. Passing the buck by saying, 'You will have to ask the doctor, sister or staff nurse' is unacceptable. Explaining that you don't know is acceptable, so is offering to find out more.

Try something like this to open up the conversation and allow the patient to express himself. 'It is hard to be definite about how long you have to live. If I had the answer right now, what would that mean for you?' A patient may reply, 'Well, I would put things in order', to which one could reply, 'Perhaps it is time to give that some serious consideration anyway'.

Questions about euthanasia (see chapter 9)

A request for euthanasia is actually a plea for better care. Most people are not keen to die earlier than they need to. The very word euthanasia should be a starting pistol sending us off as fast as we can to correct a wholly unacceptable situation (Doyle, 1999). Take all such questions or statements seriously and allow the patient time to talk. Death is always difficult and challenging so we must realise that we cannot make it all better. We will encounter much sadness, distress, disappointment, regret and guilt, in addition to the pleasures of mending relationships.

Responding to distress

It is likely that we have walked past the bed of many patients unaware of the distress that they are feeling. As we search for answers we soon realise that they are hard to find. Cassidy (1988) offers something helpful, and powerful to reflect upon:

> *Slowly I learn about the importance of powerlessness. I experience it in my life and I live with it in my work. The secret is not to be afraid of it — not to run away. The dying know we are not God... All they ask is that we do not desert them.*

Think carefully about this statement. Cassidy tells us that sharing a difficult question is more important than answering it if our patients are to feel cared for rather than deserted. Communicating with patients and families is not about having all the answers and fixing all problems. First and foremost, we must learn to distinguish between the fixable and the unfixable. Communicating is about sharing the journey, the darkness and the light.

The words of Henri Nouwen (1986) offer a thought-provoking guide to how we can help those in distress:

> *When we honestly ask ourselves which person in our lives means the most to us, we often find that it is those who, instead of giving much advice, solutions, or cures, have chosen rather to share our pain and touch our wounds with a gentler and tender hand.*

> *The friend who can be silent with us in a moment of despair and confusion, who can stay with us in our hour of grief and bereavement, who can tolerate not knowing, not curing, not healing and face with us the reality of our powerlessness, that is a friend who cares.*

Think about what it would be like if you were living with an advancing illness like cancer, MND, HIV, or heart disease. If you had to describe your communication needs what would they be? They would probably include:

- information about your illness, how it will affect you, and how to cope with it
- honesty
- professionals who talk to each other
- someone to listen to you
- someone to be with you but not to talk
- every day conversation about what is happening in the world
- opportunities to say goodbye
- companionship
- love and affection.

Timely and open communication is a cornerstone of palliative care. Without effective communication pain and symptom control cannot be achieved, no matter how much knowledge we have about the latest drugs.

Communication is not and never has been a simple process and one must remember that it takes place within highly complex social systems. Although we have considered some of the mechanisms and attitudes required to facilitate effective communication, it would be presumptuous to suggest that it is as simple as learning a set of skills. In addition to learning skills, attention must be paid to the complex relationships where you work.

Responding to patients and their families

We become adept at social chat and, to some extent, giving factual information. Unfortunately, we sometimes enter into collusion with relatives and develop techniques which block rather than facilitate meaningful discussion. Cooley (2000) explains how to guide your conversations so that they are based more on facilitating than on blocking.

Blocking tactics, include:

- ☺ changing the subject
- ☺ inappropriate information
- ☺ selective attention (to physical but not psychological factors)
- ☺ normalising or belittling comments
- ☺ premature false reassurance
- ☺ leading, closed and multiple questions
- ☺ passing the buck
- ☺ changing focus to the relatives
- ☺ jollying along and personal chit chat.

Blocking — some examples:

Patient: *I feel awful today, I think I'll stay in bed this morning.*

Nurse: *Come on now don't be a lazy bones, it's a lovely day outside.*

Patient: *I am finding it very difficult to sleep.*

Nurse: *Mmm, and how's your appetite?*

Patient: *This is much worse than I thought it would be.*

Nurse: *And how is your wife coping?*

Patient: *This wound is very sore when I move.*

Nurse: *Yes, everybody finds that.*

Patient: *How do you think I am getting on nurse?*

Nurse: *Have you asked the doctor?*

Facilitation techniques — be aware of your skills

- ☺ let the patient speak
- ☺ listening
- ☺ acknowledging
- ☺ picking up cues
- ☺ open questions
- ☺ warmth and empathy
- ☺ clarification
- ☺ confrontation
- ☺ information
- ☺ repetition and reiteration
- ☺ conversation encouragers, eg. nodding, smiling, touch
- ☺ paraphrasing and reflecting
- ☺ talk about feelings, emotions and distress
- ☺ manage silences carefully without being tempted to rush in
- ☺ be tentative.

Facilitating techniques — some examples

Patient: *I feel awful today, I think I'll stay in bed this morning.*

Nurse: *That's not like you John...What do you mean when you say awful?*

Patient: *I am finding it very difficult to sleep.*

Nurse: *That must be distressing, is there anything I can do to help?*

Patient: *This is much worse than I thought it would be.*

Nurse: *What is it that you feel is so bad?*

Patient: *This wound is very sore when I move.*

Nurse: *Let's have a look; I am sure there is something I can do to help.*

Patient: *How do you think I am getting on nurse?*

Nurse: *There seems to be something worrying you, would you like to tell me about it?*

Aim for more ☺ and less ☹!
Be alert for awkward questions, they are often heavily disguised.

Patient: *Do you get many patients in here with this?*
Nurse 1: *Oh yes, we had twenty-three last month, Mr Jones is a specialist you know.*
Nurse 2: *You look a little worried; I'm not sure why you ask that question.*

Check
it out!

A word about euphemisms

The English language in general and healthcare language in particular is full of euphemisms. Death, dying and cancer has its own language which can seriously hamper effective communication. For example:

❖ **Cancer:** Something nasty, something awful, the big one, the big C, the crab, etc.

❖ **Death and dying:** Gone, gone to sleep, gone to heaven, gone to be with the angels, passed away, passed on, passed over, etc.

It is essential that we are crystal clear when we are communicating with patients and their families, as the following examples show:

Nurse: *I am very sorry but Bill has jut gone* (meaning Bill is dead)

Bill's wife: *OK nurse, I'll nip to the shops and call in when he comes back.*

Patient: *Nurse, how long do you think I have got?* (meaning how long before I go to theatre).

Nurse: *Mmm, err, well it's too soon to say I think we will have to wait until you come back.*

Conclusion

> *Wisdom is the reward you get for a lifetime of listening when you'd have preferred to talk.*
>
> (Source unknown)

Palliative care is based on the firm foundation of sensitive, open communication between patients, families and professionals. Despite successive reports identifying weaknesses throughout healthcare systems, it is possible to provide the kind of care our patients need and deserve. The future of healthcare is in your hands. Grasp it and carry it with care and compassion.

References

Anstey S (1991) Communication. In: Penson J, Fisher R, eds. *Palliative Care for People with Cancer*. Edward Arnold, London

Booth R (2000) Spirituality: Sharing the journey. In: Cooper J,ed. *Stepping into Palliative Care. A handbook for community professionals*. Radcliffe Medical Press, Oxford

Buckman R (1988) *I Don't Know What To Say... How to help and support someone who is dying*. Papermac, Basingstoke

Buckman R (1992) *How To Break Bad News: A guide for health care professionals*. Papermac, Basingstoke

Cassidy S (1988) *Sharing the Darkness: The spirituality of caring*. Darton Longman, and Todd Limited, London: chap 8

Cooley C (2000) Communication skills in palliative care. *Prof Nurse* **15**(9): 6603–05

Covey S (1989) *The Seven Habits of Highly Effective People*. Simon and Schuster, London

Department of Health (2000) *The NHS Cancer Plan: A plan for investment, A plan for reform*. HMSO, London

Doyle D (1999) *The Platform Ticket. Memories and musing of a hospice doctor*. Pentland Press, Edinburgh

Grove V (1999) Why the NHS must spend on palliative care. *The Times* 10 June 1999: 21

Jones A (1999) A heavy and blessed experience: a psychoanalytical study of community Macmillan nurses and their role in serious illness and palliative care. *J Adv Nurs* **30**(6) :1297–1303

Nouwen HJM (1986) *Out of Solitude*. Walker and Company, New York

Rowling JK (1997) *The Philosopher's Stone*. Bloomsbury Publications, London

Twycross R (1995) *Introducing Palliative Care*. Radcliffe Medical Press, Oxford: 17–33

Useful websites

The Plain English Campaign
http://www.plainenglish.co.uk/

Chapter links to the NMC's *Code of Professional Conduct* (2002)

2. Respect the patient or client as an individual
    2.1 Partnership in care.
    2.2 Promote and respect dignity.
    2.4 Help patient's gain access to information and support.

3. Obtain consent before you give any treatment or care
    3.1 The right to information.
    3.2 Respect for autonomy.

4. Cooperate with others in the team
    4.3 Communicate your skill, knowledge and expertise.
    4.4 Ensure accurate record keeping.

6. Maintain your professional knowledge and competence
    6.4 Facilitate the learning of others.
    6.5 Deliver care based on evidence, research and best practice.

Chapter 9

Ethical issues

Once upon a time a patient died and went to heaven, but was not certain of where he was. Puzzled, he asked a nurse who was standing by his bedside: 'Nurse, am I dead?' To which she replied: 'Have you asked your doctor?'

Edwards, 1983

The overriding message from this rather tongue in cheek quotation is a simple one: there is a need, moreso now than ever before, for nurses to have the knowledge and skills to make difficult ethical decisions. No longer can nurses abrogate responsibility for this to their medical colleagues who, in reality, are little better equipped or educated than nurses in this complex, dynamic and sensitive area of health care (House of Lords Report, 1994).

Ethical decision-making is rarely about major life threatening issues in daily practice, but about being treated decently, being listened to, setting acceptable standards and responding to others in a reciprocal way. This chapter will not enter into a detailed debate surrounding the many and complex approaches to ethics, but will concern itself with the main guiding principles that help support the practical reality of behaving ethically with the dying and their family in whatever setting care is delivered.

Ethical principles in health care

There are four simple ethical principles which need to be understood when considering the decisions that are made by healthcare professionals about end of life issues. The codes of conduct and guidelines for practice that exist for many professions including nursing are underpinned by these four principles (Beauchamp and Childress, 1994).

Beneficence

Doing good for others. The duty to do good and to prevent harm and to act in the best interest of the client.

Non-maleficence

The duty to do no harm. Any intervention needs to be weighed against the good and the bad effects.

Justice

As applied to the person's rights, what the person deserves according to their needs.

Respect for autonomy

The freedom to determine one's own future without external constraints. It relies upon truth telling, accurate information, varying value systems and understanding.

If you refer to your copy of the Nursing and Midwifery Council's *Code of Professional Conduct* (2002) you will be able to cross-reference these principles throughout much of the document.

What influences decision-making?

- the law
- local policies and protocols
- professional codes of conduct
- others: the group I am working with
- past experience
- conscience
- the consequences of my actions
- the influence I have
- support from others (perceived and actual)
- culture and religion
- upbringing and education
- energy and drive
- relationship to the person(s) or issues.

Skills/approaches that are useful when dealing with ethical issues

⌘ *Acknowledgement of beliefs, values, prejudice and feelings:* This is an easy statement to make, but requires a high degree of reflective maturity.

⌘ *Involving others:* There is a clear obligation to work collaboratively with other members of the healthcare team where difficult decisions are needed. This is a key component of the NMC *Code of Professional Conduct* and essential for informed decision-making.

⌘ *Information:* Gain as much as possible from as many sources as possible: Each situation is unique in the context of the circumstances presented; a sound knowledge of such is essential.

⌘ *Standards/protocols:* As well as relevant codes of conduct, local policies should always be referred to for specific advice.

⌘ *Finding out the needs of patients, relatives:* A core component of the palliative approach to care is to find out and respond to the patients' issues as they perceive them.

⌘ *Negotiating skills:* The need for tact, diplomacy, good active listening skills and a non-judgmental, objective approach has never been greater in our increasingly litigious society.

⌘ *Humility to learn from our experience:* A willingness to acknowledge our limitations and to actively learn from the rich experiences we encounter, no matter the outcome, and to maintain an intelligent self-respect.

Some of the key ethical issues in palliative care today

- collusion,
- 'Do not resuscitate' orders
- advance directives (living wills)
- hydration close to death
- double effect
- extraordinary *vs* futile treatments
- withdrawal of treatment
- hastening death
- passive/active interventions.

There are a number of useful well-developed frameworks available to assist in decision making which have been well published and evaluated in clinical practice. Perhaps the most well known is Seedhouse's ethical grid (1988). This four-layer grid enables different aspects of an ethical issue to be worked through in a logical manner.

> ❖ The central layer looks at respect, autonomy and the person's needs and is at the core of any decision that is made.
> ❖ The second layer considers deontological (duty) issues, such as intent, doing good, minimizing harm and truth telling.
> ❖ The third layer considers consequentialist issues (the consequences of an action) and asks the question how will this benefit the individual, a group of people in similar circumstances, and society.
> ❖ The fourth layer considers the external forces influencing care such as those listed earlier.

Each of these layers is seen as independent, yet all clearly have a strong relationship with one another.

Another is Greipp's model (1992) which was developed to take account of the complex social, legal and economic factors which affect healthcare decisions today. This model places the same core ethical principles centrally and puts nursing and patient influences on either side. It emphasises the importance of existing knowledge, culture, education and our own personal beliefs on our professional practice. It could be argued that this perspective on ethical decision-making is more in tune with contemporary nursing practice, in that it more closely recognises everyday realities.

Niebuhr's model, however, which was developed in the 1960s (Tschudin, 1994) brings in the element of intuition to ethical decisions and, in the context of palliative care, would seem entirely appropriate. This model asks the reader to work through a problem by answering a series of questions.

> ❖ What is happening now? (based on your gut feeling)
> ❖ What would happen if? (certain actions were taken)
> ❖ After careful thought what is the most appropriate answer?
> ❖ What has been the end result of this action?

The simplicity of this approach is appealing to many, particularly as it embraces the abstract element of intuition that is so cherished by nurses in practice. There is still a need to consider the four core ethical principles discussed at the beginning of the chapter and to bring in the influences of professional codes and duty.

No single model will suit all occasions and to offer specific advice on each possible scenario encountered would be impossible; but the important link between ethics and caring has to be the central focus of any decisions made in ethical situations. Nurses have a distinct advantage, in that, while nursing does not have a monopoly on caring approaches, it is the single most important underpinning principle that defines the profession itself.

The principle of double effect

One of the most controversial and frequently misunderstood aspects of pain control in terminal care is the effect that high doses of opiates have on the patient close to death. There is an increasing body of evidence, which dispels the popular myth that respiratory depression is an inevitable consequence of opiate usage in the terminally ill (Bercovitch *et al*, 1999; Morita *et al*, 2001; Fohr, 1998). Unfortunately, this stance is used all too often by inexperienced doctors and nurses — who are worried about the possible consequences of hastening a patient's death — to justify not prescribing appropriate dose titrated to the patients' needs. The consequence of this for the patient is that frequently their pain remains uncontrolled up to the moment of death. Something that cannot be ethically justified when the means for relieving distress is readily available.

Double effect is a well established and accepted doctrine in British law (R *v* Adams 1957 [randall and Downie, 1996]) and enables a doctor safely to make a decision regarding the possible effects of drugs he or she may use to help control pain and difficult symptoms, as long as the primary intention of the drug prescribed is to relieve distress, hence the term double effect. In simple terms, it asks the question, 'what is the intention here'. It also reflects the important moral principles of; (a) doing good for your patient and, (b) acting in the patient's best interest.

Advance directives

The advance directive is an American concept which has been adapted and used in the UK in a limited way for some twenty years now. It is based around the very simple idea that a person can leave instructions about their possible medical treatment, in case there comes a time when they are no longer capable of making decisions or of communicating them.

What does it do? Many people fear that, if they become ill, they could face a situation where they may be given too much treatment when there is little or no chance of recovery, or given treatment which would leave them in a condition with which they could not cope. A living will can show that in the future, under clearly defined circumstances, the patient does not want treatment which will help him or her to live longer, such as antibiotics, tube feeding or being kept alive indefinitely on a life support machine. It is important to recognise that advance directives are an entirely separate issue from voluntary euthanasia, and should not be confused with the debate about assisted dying.

Is it legally binding? Although there is no law that governs the use of living wills, in common law refusing treatment beforehand is legal as long as it meets the following conditions:

⌘ The person is mentally able, is not suffering any mental distress and is over eighteen when he or she makes the request.

⌘ The person was fully informed about the nature and consequence of the living will at the time he or she made it.

⌘ The person is clear that the living will should apply to all situations or circumstances which arise later.

⌘ The person is not pressurised or influenced by anyone else when he or she made the decision.

⌘ The living will has not been changed either verbally or in writing since it was drawn up.

⌘ The person is now mentally incapable of making any decision because they are unconscious or otherwise unfit.

There are now a small but significant number of UK case law precedents that have sought both to challenge advance directives and to endorse them. It is becoming increasingly clear that they do have legal validity, provided that the conditions are adhered to.

What are the advantages and disadvantages? When a medical team is faced with a difficult decision about what treatment or care to give to a patient who is not able to make a decision, a living will helps the team to know what the patient would have wanted if he or she had been conscious. However, the advance directive will still have to be interpreted to make sure that the situation it describes does still apply to the patient. Apart from allowing the patient to control the treatment he or she receives, the living will also gives the patient the opportunity to discuss difficult issues with close family and friends.

What do I do if I come across one? If you should be made aware of an advance directive's existence by a patient or relative, inform the person in charge. The document does not have to be kept by a solicitor and can be kept in the patient's notes. All members of the healthcare team should be made aware of its contents and provided the conditions, as outlined above, are clear, it now has growing legal validity.

The law in the UK is evolving slowly to take account of living wills and there is a growing body of case law to inform decisions in this area. The British Medical Association, the Patient's Association, the Royal College of Nursing and the Government have all confirmed that they support living wills. The Royal College of Nursing have issued some clear and helpful guidance for nurses and the document itself can be downloaded from the RCN website.

'Do not resuscitate' orders

Few areas of health care cause as much confusion amongst nurses as this contentious issue. What is not in question here is a cardiac arrest affecting a previously healthy individual. The law is clear cut, they should be treated until it is obvious that they cannot survive the arrest and a doctor decides resuscitation measures should cease. The NMC's *Code of Professional Conduct* (2002) endorses this view entirely. The concern is what should happen to those people who have a known diagnosis and whose illness is liable to end in death, and if cardiopulmonary resuscitation (CPR) were to be attempted which would seriously affect their remaining quality of life.

In response to growing public and professional concern the RCN and BMA issued a joint statement in 2001 to offer up-to-date guidance for practitioners. It concludes that:

Guiding principles

⌘ Timely support for patients and people close to them and effective, sensitive communication are essential.
⌘ Decisions must be based on the individual patient's circumstances and reviewed regularly.
⌘ Sensitive advance discussion should always be encouraged, but not forced.
⌘ Information about CPR and the chances of a successful outcome needs to be realistic.

Issues for consideration: competent adults

Information giving

⌘ Ensure patient has access to information about decision making in relation to CPR.

Discussion

⌘ Senior health professionals should initiate sensitive discussion with the patient.

⌘ Respect the patient's wish not to discuss resuscitation.

Assess the clinical issues

⌘ Is CPR likely to restart the patient's heart and breathing?

⌘ Would restarting the patient's heart and breathing provide any benefit?

⌘ Do the expected benefits outweigh the potential burdens of treatment?

Seek consensus

⌘ Responsibility for the decision rests with the consultant or GP in charge of care.

⌘ Record patient's wishes clearly in notes and communicate decision to relevant health professionals.

Issues for consideration: incompetent adults

Is there a valid and applicable advance refusal of CPR?

Proxy decision makers (Scotland only)

⌘ Consult any appointed proxy decision maker and follow procedures in Adults with Incapacity (Scotland) Act.

Assess the best interests of the patient

⌘ What is known about the patient's wishes regarding resuscitation?

⌘ Did the patient request confidentiality?

⌘ Did the patient identify people to be consulted about treatment?

⌘ Seek the views of people close to the patient about what he or she would want.

⌘ Discuss with the clinical team.

The assessment of clinical issues remains the same as with competent adults.

Euthanasia

This is perhaps the most emotive, misunderstood and controversial of all the ethical issues to face in health care today. This subject raises an immensely complex set of arguments which embrace society's core values and, potentially, its future laws. It is for this reason that it is hotly debated in the media and continually discussed by professionals. We all have a vested interest in getting it right, because decisions regarding our own health and welfare in future years may well rest on how society views purposeful and deliberate, medical assistance to end life.

There are numerous definitions of euthanasia, which in many ways only serve to add to the confusion, but however it is defined, the key moral and ethical issues are; (a) the intention or motive behind the act itself and, (b) the consequences for that individual and society as a whole. This chapter will not enter into a debate around these issues, nor concern itself with the rapidly changing international scene, but will simply attempt to give an overview of the current legal and ethical advice that is available.

The position for all healthcare staff regarding euthanasia is abundantly clear in British law. Even though they may morally sympathise with a patient's wishes to die and be witness to physical suffering that cannot be fully controlled by modern pharmacological intervention, they are prohibited by criminal law to take any steps or give any advice to the patient or, indeed, the relatives to help them carry out that wish (Dimond, 1995).

The principles of euthanasia are based on the assumption that some people, because of their circumstances, are 'better off dead', and their lives are 'not worth living'. Also, that we should treat them in the same way as we would treat a sick animal. That principle simply pays no heed to whether the death is voluntary or involuntary. British law is founded on the idea that all human life has equal value and is entitled to protection. There is no better way to undermine this principle than to agree that some people, albeit in difficult circumstances, have the right to ask others to assist them to die, because the person concerned agrees that they are better off dead.

The RCN the BMA have both issued advice on this subject and copies of the documents can be found on the websites listed at the end of the chapter. There is little empirically gained advice of a pragmatic nature, however, within the abundance of literature that has been written on this subject, two authors that do attempt to offer advice are Voigt (1995) and Cole (1993). Both articles are based on the authors work with HIV patients.

Cole (1993) cites four case studies which demonstrate widely varying reasons for requesting euthanasia and attempts to give caregivers some ideas about how to respond to these requests. To do so, he considers that they need to suspend their own feelings about the morality of a request for euthanasia and be able to acknowledge the reality of the pain that has led a patient to ask to die. He proposes:

- ask the patient about it
- acknowledge the request as sincere
- investigate the reasons
- correct the correctable
- return control to the patient
- think about the spiritual dimension
- admit your own powerlessness.

Voigt (1995) adopts a similar stance, but proposes his own systematic strategy, ie:

- determining the patient's fears
- evaluating the risk of depression
- determining expectations
- establishing support networks
- discussing the options and plans available.

Neither author offers a definitive solution and rightly point out the need for an individualistic approach which is patient-centred. There have been six attempts since the Second World War to obtain legislation legalising euthanasia in this country, and each time the proposed bill has been overwhelmingly defeated in parliament at the first vote. The House of Lords have recently debated this issue once more and, in the near future, it is possible that a further attempt at permissive legislation will be forthcoming (House of Lords, 2003). There will always be those people in any society that make a conscious and rational decision to end their life. That is a legitimate choice, albeit regrettable. What we, as a society, have to decide is whether we are prepared to take the risk of passing legislation for that minority to allow others to assist them, potentially at the expense of undermining the care that is offered to the significant majority.

The ethics of hydration

Nurses have an ethical duty to recognise and treat malnutrition in competent patients as part of optimal care and this is usually attended to by eating and drinking. There is an increasing realisation, however, that artificial hydration of the terminally ill, where it is clearly recognised that the patient is dying and they are not capable of receiving oral nutrition, is not a good idea. Ethical problems arise where tube feeding is in place which permits the maintenance of tissue metabolism even though a patient cannot eat anything. This is an active medical treatment which demands good consultation, through the whole healthcare team, as to when it is started, stopped or continued in the long term for incompetent patients (Lennard Jones, 1998)

Questions nurses need to ask themselves

⌘ What are (or what would you expect to be) the overall effects of hydration on this patient? Does the patient appear to 'feel better' as a result of the infusion? Is their well being enhanced?

⌘ Is there any reason to believe that specific symptoms are being relieved by artificial hydration.

⌘ Are some symptoms being aggravated? If so, which?

⌘ Is the IV infusion improving the patient's alertness? If so, is this what the patient wants?

⌘ Does it appear that the infusion may be prolonging the patient's survival? If so, is this in keeping with their preferences?

⌘ What are the psychosocial effects? Is the infusion interfering with family interactions?

⌘ Is family stress increased?

Zerwekh, 1987

The nurses role in terminal hydration

⌘ Establish whether the patient has an advance directive.

⌘ Reassure the patient and family that at all times the comfort of the patient is paramount. Wilkes (1994) reminds us that we must be tactfully resistant to sacrificing the interests of the patient to the emotional distress of the relatives.

⌘ Always present facts carefully, explain fully the benefits and burdens.

⌘ Ensure excellent holistic care is given at all times.

⌘ Early discussion with the patient and family to determine the patient's wishes.

⌘ Give regular mouth care, offer ice cubes and sips of water if tolerated. Provide cream for lips to prevent cracking. Encourage the family to help provide this care.

⌘ Ensure pain relief is adequate — reassess regularly.

⌘ Give good pressure area care, keep the patient clean and dry at all times.

⌘ Listen and support the patient at all times. Remember that they trust us.

⌘ Reassure the family that stopping IV fluids is not stopping care.
⌘ Remember that using the palliative approach in an acute setting is not an excuse for bad practice. Where time and staffing resources are short we need to make sure that we keep very closely involved in patient care when they no longer need acute interventions.

Overall, it is likely that patients and relatives will increasingly expect good nutritional care as part of medical treatment to prolong life and improve quality of life, this is their right. It is also likely that the public will increasingly come to accept that hydration or nutrition via a tube should not be used when it impairs the dignity and comfort of those who are dying.

The Law and palliative care

There is no single terminal care act on the statute books in the UK that governs how to approach the dying from a legal perspective. Case precedent and history provide the basis for most law concerning end of life issues; and with the numerous high profile cases that have made the media headlines over the last few years, the public are becoming much more aware of these issues.

What needs to be remembered is that case law is underpinned by four principles:

❖ Treatment cannot be given without consent.
❖ There is no automatic right to treatment.
❖ There is no right to active assisted death.
❖ Intent needs to be clear.

When caring for patients who are terminally ill we must:

❖ Make sure that the person is dying and this is acknowledged by the whole healthcare team.
❖ Be certain of our motives, be explicit in our explanations, discuss it with the healthcare team, and accurately record it at all stages.
Potential issues include:

❖ The person's understanding of the nature of the treatment.
❖ Their understanding of the purpose and effects of the treatment.
❖ Their ability to retain this information.

References

Beauchamp TL, Childress JF (1994) *Principles of Biomedical Ethics*. 4th edn. Oxford University Press, Oxford

Bercovitch M, Waller A, Adunsky A (1999) High dose morphine use in the hospice setting: A database survey of patient characteristics and effect on life expectancy. *Cancer* **86**: 871–7

Nursing and Midwifery Council (2002) *Code of Professional Conduct*. NMC, London

British Medical Association, the Resuscitation Council (UK) and the Royal College of Nursing (2001) *Decisions relating to Cardiopulmonary Resuscitation*. BMA, Resuscitation Council and the RCN: February

Dimond B (1995) *Legal aspects of Nursing*. Prentice Hall, Hemel Hempstead

Cole RM (1993) Communicating with people who request euthanasia. *Palliative Med* **7**: 139–43

Edwards P (1983) Am I going to die nurse? *Nurs Times* **79**(10): 27–8

Fohr SA (1998) The double effect of pain medication: Separating myth from reality. *J Pall Med* **1**(4): 315–28

Greipp M (1992) Greipps' model of ethical decision making. *J Adv Nurs* **17**: 734–8

House of Lords (1994) *Report of the Select Committee on Medical Ethics*. HMSO, London

House of Lords (2003) Patient Assisted Dying Bill (Bill 37) The Lord Joffe. HMSO, London

Lennard Jones JE (1998) *Ethical and Legal Aspects of Clinical Hydration and Nutritional Support*. Report for the British Association for Parenteral and Enteral Nutrition

Morita T, Tsunoda J, Inoue S, Chihara S (2001) Effects of high dose opioids and sedatives on survival in terminally ill cancer patients. *J Pain Symptom Management* **21**: 282–9

Randall F, Downie RS (1996) Regina v Adams 1957. Cited in: *Palliative Care Ethics A Good Companion*. Oxford University Press, New York: chap 4

Seedhouse D (1988) *Ethics: The heart of health care*. John Wiley, Chichester

Tschudin V (1994) *Deciding Ethically*. Baillière Tindall, London

Voigt RF (1995) Euthanasia and HIV disease: How can physicians respond? *J Palliative Care* **11**(2): 38–41

Wilkes E (1994) On withholding nutrition and hydration in the terminally ill: has palliative medicine gone too far? A commentary. *J Med Ethics* **20**: 144–5

Zerwekh JV (1987) Should fluid and nutritional support be withheld from terminally ill patients. *Am J Hospice Care* **4**(4): 37–8

Useful websites

The British Medical Association
http://web.bma.org.uk/ap.nsf/Content/__Hub+ethics

MedEthex online
http://griffin.mcphu.edu/MedEthEx/intro.html

The International Association for Hospice and Palliative Care
http://www.hospicecare.com/Ethics/ethics.htm

StopPain.Org
http://www.stoppain.org/palliative_care/ethics.html

BBC Ethics Home Page
http://www.bbc.co.uk/religion/ethics/sanctity_life/euthpallcare.shtml

National Hospice Council
(http://www.hospice-spc-council.org.uk)

Royal College of Nursing — go to witnessing resuscitation guidelines for nursing staff
http://www.rcn.org.uk/members/publications/

Chapter links to the NMC's *Code of Professional Conduct* (2002)

All clauses and sub clauses of the *Code of Professional Conduct* are relevant to good ethical nursing practice, but it is useful to highlight one that is new and directly relevant to this chapter.

3.6. Competency and advance statements

This clause mentions advance statements for the first time within the code and talks of the need to find out any previously indicated preferences in treatment when the patient is no longer competent.

Chapter 10

Spiritual care

> The old grey donkey Eeyore stood by himself in a thistly corner of the forest, his front feet well apart, his head on one side and thought about things. Sometimes he thought sadly to himself 'Why?' and sometimes he thought 'Where?' and sometimes he didn't quite know what he was thinking about.
>
> AA Milne, 1992

If, like Eeyore, you have ever asked yourself the questions 'why me? why this? and why now?' in the midst of a life crisis (and for certain we all have) then it may surprise you to know that it could be argued that you were in some way being spiritual. Whether you have a formal belief that guides your life, or not, we all need to find meaning and perspective to major events in our lives and there is no greater life crisis than facing our mortality. It is this that makes spiritual care such an important and integral concept in all nursing practice, but it is particularly focused in a palliative care context.

Nursing literature offers a wide variety of definitions of both spirituality and religion, and for the most part there is agreement that the relationship between spirituality and conventional religious belief is confused and ambiguous. It is hardly surprising that most nurses find interpreting and delivering such a sensitive area of nursing care a major challenge. Indeed, McSherry and Draper (1997) argue that to address spirituality adequately, nurses need to be self-aware, mature and introspective. They comment that these elements are a major barrier since individuals will need to explore areas of their lives that are sacred, private and deeply personal. Equally, Kristeller *et al* (1999) argues that the majority of general nurses feel that spiritual issues are neglected because of time constraints, a lack of confidence in managing these issues and role uncertainty.

It has also been argued that fear may be a reason for nurses' reluctance to incorporate spiritual care into practice: fear of getting into a situation that they cannot handle; fear of intruding on a patient's privacy; and fear of being converted or confused in their own belief system (Granstrom, 1990).

It is certainly true that nurses generally find spiritual health care hard to articulate because it raises so many questions about life in which there are no specific answers or probable certainties, and part of the problem is perhaps rooted in the language used to describe spiritual care and needs. By its very nature it is inherently profound, philosophical, sometimes religious in orientation and, almost invariably, ancient in its foundation. It is often both unfamiliar and difficult language for many people to use in conversation, especially at times of stress.

Becker (2001) argues that we should perhaps be trying to develop a more appropriate and acceptable vocabulary that represents spirituality as a caring concept. A vocabulary that is representative of contemporary language with the use of metaphors and phrases that don't induce the 'cringe' factor and without the use of slang or colloquialisms. This would not only help patients and families, it would also help the professionals who work with the dying in whatever setting, as they themselves find it just as difficult to understand and approach spiritual matters due, in part, to the vocabulary (Ross, 1994).

Despite these acknowledged difficulties, there is clear evidence to suggest that the meeting of spiritual needs can improve the physical well being of patients (Waugh, 1992). Many patients also state that attention to the spiritual side of their life adds to their well being and can even counteract some of the more negative aspects of illness (Catterall, 1998).

There is a common misconception that to meet spiritual needs a nurse needs either to have a religious belief themselves, or to have undergone some special training to deliver complicated interventions (Kemp, 1994). The reality, according to Ross (1996), is that there was no evidence to suggest that nurses who had been taught spiritual care were any better at doing it. It appears that the personal characteristics of the nurse seemed to determine the spiritual care they gave.

The simple but emphatic message is that spiritual care is an integral and vital aspect of all nurses' work in whatever setting, but is particularly focused with the dying who, regardless of culture, belief or background are common in their search for a meaningful context to the crushing emotional and physical dilemmas posed by terminal illness.

No formal definition of spiritual care will be offered in this book for the reasons stated at the beginning of this chapter; however, it is appropriate to share with you one of the simplest and most understandable statements ever uttered in this context to help you to gain a clear sense of perspective. These words come direct from the mouth of Cannon Ian Ainsworth Smith who is a Chaplain at a major London teaching hospital. When asked for his own interpretation of spirituality and care he said:

Spiritual care... can help provide either a lot of answers to profound questions, or provide a context in which a person can safely ask lots of difficult questions. There are not necessarily any answers, but we can learn to stay with the questions. Spiritual care can be described as how someone puts together your past, your present, and any future life you may have and what this means to you.

Nurses are frequently polarised in their approaches to the spiritual dimension and tend to adopt one or other of the following viewpoints:

- ⌘ Spiritual care will be defined as a purely psychosocial problem where all 'so called' spiritual needs can be explained by reference to psychological and sociological theory.
- ⌘ The existence of any concept which considers spirituality is denied totally and patient needs defined in this way are avoided.
- ⌘ Acknowledge the relevance of caring for the spirit as an important part of care, worthy of independent theory and consideration.

> Ask yourself which you subscribe to and why?

Our patients, however, are facing the reality of their own mortality and can find the challenge of searching for meaning very difficult, for example:

- ⌘ A person who has placed their faith in modern science and medicine to provide the answers, will feel let down and disappointed when told 'We cannot cure you'.
- ⌘ A person who has lived their life doing good for others and who has a strong faith, believing that God will reward them, can have their faith undermined by the experience of enduring a difficult and potentially terminal illness.
- ⌘ A person whose philosophy tells them that the material world is all that there is, and when its your turn to die, that's it, is surprised when he finds himself saying 'Why me? What does it all mean?' and, 'Is there something more?'

Case study: Harry

Harry is sixty-three years old, married with three grown up children. He is a fork lift truck driver in a local factory and has a strong Christian faith. He has a diagnosis of carcinoma of the lung and is being treated with radiotherapy in the oncology ward of his local hospital. A student goes to his bedside one morning and he angrily says to her, 'Why me? Why has God let this happen to me?' He is bitter towards life in general and also towards the members of his church community where he has been a lay reader for some years, as no one has come to visit him.

How can you help address the spiritual needs of someone like Harry? Here is a suggested strategy.

Problem:	Spiritual distress and anger due to questioning of his faith
Care plan:	Build trust and rapport with Harry.
	Listen carefully to his anxieties and encourage him to talk about his needs.
	Adopt a non-judgmental and empathic approach
	Ask his permission to contact the clergy in charge of his church to arrange a visit
	Ask if he wishes to see the hospital chaplain.

Spiritual needs are universal to humankind and can include the need:

- to love and to be loved
- to achieve a sense of purpose and meaning in our life
- to keep a sense of identity, individual value and worth
- to maintain a sense of realistic hope in life
- to fulfil relationships with people who matter to us
- to express our personal sexuality in terms of appearance
- to value the importance of truth, freedom and responsibility
- to engage in meaningful work
- to be creative in our life
- to enjoy abstract, aesthetic pleasures which give personal meaning.

Ask yourself how many of these apply in your life at the moment?

Religious needs are specific to those people who have a definitive faith and can include the need:

- for individual and corporate worship
- to engage in personal and corporate prayer
- to take part in birth, maturation, marriage and death rituals
- for meditation and private contemplation
- to see a religious person who represents their faith
- to visit holy places

- to possess holy items which assist in the expression of faith
- to follow a religious vocation if desired.

> Ask yourself how many of these apply in
> your life at the moment?

Many patients express their spiritual pain by asking seemingly impossible questions. These are questions which are mostly rhetorical in nature, and do not necessarily demand an explanatory response. Questions like:

~ *How will I die?*
~ *Will I be alone?*
~ *Will I suffer?*
~ *Why me?*
~ *Is my illness some sort of punishment?*
~ *I can't understand how I am feeling*
~ *Am I behaving as I should?*
~ *Is there a god at all?*
~ *I don't have a faith?*
~ *Am I being a hypocrite looking for god's help?*
~ *Will anyone take me seriously?*
~ *Will people tell me the truth?*

If you have ever encountered these questions and stayed with a patient trying to support them, you have delivered spiritual care. You may well have walked away feeling inadequate, unsure as to whether you have helped the person or not. Below are some suggested questions to ask your self that are, for most of us, eminently answerable.

⌘ Have I got a basic understanding of the differences between 'agnostics, atheists, and believers'?
⌘ Do I understand what some people believe to be reincarnation?
⌘ Have I ever considered this subject myself and where do I stand?
⌘ How do I find/get meaning in my life and work?
⌘ What do I value in my life?

Here are some suggestions of questions to ask to assist in discovering a patient's spiritual needs. The list is not exhaustive, merely a guide and can be supplemented by your own questions.

~ *How have you coped with your illness up to now?*
~ *What are your thoughts while facing this difficulty?*

~ *What is the hardest part of this for you?*
~ *What else is happening in your life now?*
~ *Has being ill brought about any new insights into your life?*
~ *What is your biggest fear?*

Some more general questions that are not so direct, include:

~ *Tell me about your life?*
~ *What happened to you?*
~ *What have you done in your life that you feel good about?**
~ *What has been the happiest part of your life?*
~ *What challenges and difficulties have you had to face?*

Responding to these questions is equally difficult. Here are some reflective and empathic responses that may be appropriate:

~ *This must be really hard for you.*
~ *As I listen I can sense your distress.*
~ *Whatever you are feeling is understandable given the situation you are facing.*

Case study: Hugh

Hugh is a forty-year-old school teacher and is married with two young children. He has been admitted to hospital in the latter stages of prostate cancer. He is a quiet and reserved man who likes classical music and has no expressed faith. He is extremely worried about what will happen to his wife and children when he dies and is frustrated by his weakness and loss of independence and control over his life.

Problem:	Anxiety due to concerns over the security of his family
Care plan:	Help him to review his plans for his family and to set new goals
Problem:	Feels helpless because of his illness
Care plan:	Foster realistic hope by helping him focus on the achievements in his life and happy events that give meaning to him
	Encourage him to use his family as a source of strength
Problem:	Needs an opportunity for relaxation
Care plan:	Explore the possibility of his family bringing in a walkman or of the hospital library providing one so that he can listen to his favourite classical music

The least you need to know

A range of factors may influence spiritual care; namely, the nurse, the carer, the culture and structure of the organisation, the characteristics of the patient and the family or loved ones. There are many routes to good spiritual care, some of which are simple and within the capacity of all nurses whatever their education or background.

⌘ Stay with the person; be with them and alongside them. Know when to stop doing and start being.

⌘ Listen to them and hear the pain. Being heard and accepted in the depths of despair may lift spirits and is part of sharing with sensitivity and compassion.

⌘ Drop your own agenda because that gets in the way of unconditional care. Review your own beliefs, options and biases.

⌘ Encourage them to express their fear and anger, ie. give them permission and permit yourself also to stay.

⌘ Provide a secure and caring environment which emphasises the patient's needs as they see them as paramount.

⌘ Reassure them about physical pain with information and practical help as desired and appropriate.

⌘ Help them to spend time with those who matter to them.

⌘ Help them to spend time alone and in a peaceful environment.

⌘ Use appropriate fun and humour as patients greatly appreciate this aspect of normality.

⌘ Review and remember with photos and mementos.

⌘ Provide for religious and sacramental care with the appropriate minister for communion, prayer, confession or anointing if requested.

⌘ Remember the small, but important aesthetic things in life can make a huge difference, such as:

- inspiring music, poetry or art
- chocolate
- a delicious meal or a glass of wine
- a visit from a much loved pet
- a walk in the gardens in the sunshine
- a gift of flowers, a letter or a visit from a friend
- a beautiful view and a glorious sunset.

All nurses can recall the sense of guilt they felt when they stopped to talk with a patient in the middle of a busy shift when it seemed that a thousand jobs needed doing. Forget the guilt and next time stay with that patient a little longer, because it just may have been that brief encounter and the care you demonstrated in those moments that really made the difference. Time is always a factor cited by nurses as a reason for not being able to address spiritual needs, but it need not necessarily be dependent on time. Just like the concept of palliative care as discussed in *Chapter 1*, it is a way of thinking and an attitude of mind that communicates respect, love and understanding to another.

References

Becker R (2001) Spiritual care on the rocks. *Eur J Palliative Care* **8**(4): 136

Catterall Ra, Cox M, Greet B, Sankey J, Griffiths G (1998). The assessment and audit of spiritual care. *Int J Palliative Nurs* **4**(4): 162–8

Granstrom SL (1985) Spiritual nursing care for oncology patients. *Top Clin Nurs* **7**(1): 39–45

Kemp CE (1994) Spiritual care in terminal illness. *J Hospice Palliative Care* **11**(6): 31–6

Kristeller JL, Sheedy Z, Schilling RF (1999). I would, if l could: How oncologists and oncology nurses address spiritual distress in cancer patients. *Psycho-oncology* **8**: 451–8

McSherry W, Draper P (1997) The spiritual dimension: why the absence within nursing curricula? *Nurse Education Today* **17**: 413–7

Milne AA (1992) *The Pooh Book of Quotations*. Methuen Children's Books, London: 41

Ross LA (1994) Spiritual aspects of nursing. *J Adv Nurs* **19**(3): 439–47

Ross LA (1996) Teaching spiritual care to nurses. *Nurse Educ Today* **16**: 38–43

Waugh LA (1992) *Spiritual aspects of nursing: a descriptive study of nurses' perceptions*. Unpublished PhD thesis. Queen Margaret College, Edinburgh

Useful websites

Beliefnet
http://www.beliefnet.com

Spirituality and health
http://www.spiritualityhealth.com/newsh/items/home/item_216.html

Spirituality assessment tools
http://www.chcr.brown.edu/pcoc/Spirit.htm#Spiritual%20Well-Being%20Scale

Spirituality
http://www.spirituality.com/

Chapter links to the NMC *Code of Professional Conduct* (2002)

2. Respect the patient or client as an individual
    2.1 Partnership in care
    2.2 Promote and respect dignity

2.4 Help patient's gain access to information and support

3. Obtain consent before you give any treatment or care
    3.1 The right to information
    3.2 Respect for autonomy

5. Protect confidential information
    5.1 Respect the use of information and guard against breaches of confidentiality
    5.2 Seek patient's wishes to share information

Chapter 11

Sexuality and advancing illness

Elizabeth and Walter are both eighty-two approaching their sixtieth wedding anniversary. Walter is fit and healthy. Elizabeth has breast cancer. 'Don't let them take her away from me'. 'We have never ever been apart; I need to feel the warmth of her body next to mine'. You all think I am a dirty old man.

Introduction

Sexuality is not merely the sexual act. It has multiple meanings that are shaped and influenced by life experiences. We develop our understanding of sex and sexuality throughout life, picking up cues and influences from others and from the media. These influences lead us to develop our own conclusions about life, love, desirability, appearance and relationships. Sexuality encompasses body image, physical sexual responses, the way we perceive our appearance and attractiveness to self and others. Communication and relationships, self-image and self-esteem, and the sense of affirmation and acknowledgement that we experience from others in our everyday lives are all components of sexuality (Wells, 2002).

There is evidence to show that healthcare professionals fail to provide information and support to patients and partners when patients undergo treatment for gynaecological cancers (Juraskova et al, 2003). As many as 70% of men with prostate cancer experience sexual dysfunction (Fossa et al, 1997). Issues that should have been addressed remain unresolved when the patient is receiving palliative care, but it is never too late to perform an assessment and plan care to ease distress and suffering. It is vital to understand that the location of the primary cancer or spread is only one indicator of sexual dysfunction. The quality of the pre-existing sexual relationship between patient and partner is equally, if not, more important. Men and women who are not in a committed relationship have to face the potential trauma of rejection by a new partner who learns of their illness. Some may avoid relationships because of the fear of rejection.

It is vital to understand that sex may be important or more important to patients and their partners when they face advanced illness. Intimacy expressed through words, looks and gestures allows the expression of love.

In a bitter-sweet way it serves to remind couples of what they have together but soon will lose. Illnesses, disabilities, fears and treatments inhibit sexual contact and desire. This must be taken seriously by health professionals.

Relationships and family dynamics are highly complex and difficult to understand. Although we should always try to help we must distinguish between the fixable and unfixable. A family situation that appears intolerable to us may be acceptable to the family.

Sexuality and palliative care: a neglected subject

If we claim to provide holistic care we simply cannot ignore sexuality. Roper *et al* (1980) were responsible for alerting UK nurses to sexuality when they presented their activities of living model of nursing. One of the activities is expressing sexuality. In 1987, Savage discussed nurses, gender and sexuality in a way that established addressing sexuality as a nursing responsibility. Savage interviewed one student nurse who said

> *We use Roper's model. We go through all of them, in class, and in theory it's very good. One of those is expressing sexuality and that's important. But when it comes to doing it in class, what do you talk about? Helping women to look better after they've had their hysterectomy so their husbands will want to have sex with them? You spend ages on breathing then you get to the end of the list, dying and expressing sexuality, and how we should talk to patients and get them to express their feelings, and that's it. No-one ever does it! We write in our care plans 'Encourage questions and help patients to express their feelings and anxieties', but it's never really approached.*

Although this quotation dates back to 1987, little has changed. Many of us are comfortable with innuendo and 'adult' jokes, yet we find it hard to broach the subject with our patients and offer support and simple advice. If sexual issues and questions are raised by patients and families we feel the need to refer on to a psychosexual counsellor.

Sutherland and Gamlin (1999) discussed body image and sexuality and their implications for those receiving and providing palliative care. They offer many practical suggestions for addressing sexuality. The P-L-ISS-I-T model (Annon, 1976) is described by Sutherland and Gamlin, (1999) and Gamlin (1999). This model, although originally designed to facilitate re-adjustment following myocardial infarction, has been used in palliative care.

The P-LI-SS-I-T model of sexual readjustment.

Permission

The nurse gives permission to the patient to talk about worries or concerns. This may involve asking direct questions or being available and accessible.

Limited information

Factual general information is given about the condition and how this may affect the patient's feeling and functioning. For example, what to expect after pelvic surgery and how to cope with it.

Specific suggestions

More in-depth information may be required. A knowledge of relevant anatomy, physiology and pathology will help. Specific information relating to specific cancers will be given.

Intensive therapy

Some patients and their partners may require intensive therapy, ie. referral to a psychosexual counsellor but, if the preceding steps are followed, it is likely that most patients' needs can be met without specialist referral.

Breaking the ice

If you are able to feel comfortable dealing with the permission stage of the model you will do much to help your patients. To achieve this you must decide what to say to broach the subject and give permission. Knowing your patient and choosing your moment and setting should, 'go without saying', but they don't!

Of course it can be embarrassing to discuss sexual matters with patients. This is why we don't do it. We think that we may offend them or they may not like it. It can be equally embarrassing to discuss constipation, diarrhoea and malodorous wounds, but meticulous assessment is the precursor to effective management.

The careful use of humour can help, but sensitivity and tact are essential. Think about using one or more of the following suggested questions or statements. Please remember, they are not offered as a script. You need to use words you are comfortable with.

❖ *How are things between you and your partner?* or, *How is your relationship?* This may get you into the territory you are aiming for but may be too general.

❖ *You and your partner seem a little distant?* This is not intrusive but may unearth some helpful points.

❖ *Illness puts a strain on all aspects of a relationship. How are you coping?* Again this is indirect but offers opportunities for patients to talk if they wish.

❖ *How are things in the bedroom?* Ok if you know the patient, maybe this is too much for some patients.

❖ *Sometimes patients have worries or questions about sex. If you have any questions or concerns please feel free to ask me or any of my colleagues?* Perhaps this is a little wordy, but it is direct without being offensive.

If a patient appears embarrassed or offended simply apologise but 'leave the door open'. 'I am sorry I seem to have embarrassed you'. 'Have a think about what I said and let me know if you would like to talk about things with me or another colleague'. Many people regard sexual problems as an inevitable consequence of being ill. Partners may fear 'catching the disease', causing damage or pain to the patient.

After 'breaking the ice' you may need to go on to specific questions. For example:

❖ *Have you experienced erectile dysfunction/impotence?* Many will not understand this jargon. You may need to choose carefully other terms such as, 'getting a hard on or getting it up'. If the answer is yes you can explore this further before referring to a specialist. For example, *When did this begin? Does it happen every time? Have you any thoughts about what may be causing it?*

The next step will be to check medications to see if any may cause erectile dysfunction. The very fact that you have listened and indicated that it may be possible to do something will be enormously helpful to the patient.

❖ *Have you noticed a difference in arousal/orgasm since the operation/beginning this medication?* Again you may need to re-phrase this and say for example, 'Do you find you get turned on/climax/come?' Women may tell you about pain and dryness on intercourse. Simple explanation about lubrication may help. A physical examination may be warranted.

❖ *Is this a problem for you and/or your partner?* The patient may say, 'It is/isn't a problem for either of us'. 'It's not for me but it is for him'.

❖ *Has the treatment affected your sex-life in any way?* The patient has a chance to think about this and open up if they wish.

❖ *Have you talked to your partner about how you feel?* Patients and partners experience major difficulties in talking about sex, despite a wealth of magazines and television programmes. If the answer is 'no', you and/or a colleague can offer to help by being with the patient or helping them to choose the words to open the conversation.

Confidentiality

Think very carefully about sharing intimate discussions with colleagues. Of course, teamwork is a core theme in palliative care but it may not be necessary to share this information with the entire team. Sadly, some staff do not have a mature attitude to sexuality. Inappropriate comments will undo your achievements. You must discuss findings with a qualified colleague, but choose wisely.

Sexuality and intimacy but what about love?

One word frees us from all the weight and pain in life, that word is love. (Sophocles)

I may not be smart; Jenny, but I know what love is. (Forrest Gump)

Sex is not always an expression of love, it serves many other purposes. In the context of palliative care it is vital to see its place in a loving relationship and, one which is, will be ended by the death of the patient. Find a way to use the word love in conversations with patients and families. 'I can tell he really loves you', 'When did you first fall in love?' It may cause those you care for to think long and hard about the life that is left.

Issues surrounding sexuality are, and will remain, deeply private, but if we are to deliver truly holistic palliative care we must provide an environment where patients and their partners feel able to express their concerns in the knowledge that they will be met with skill, tact, diplomacy and confidentiality. The future of this type of care is firmly in your hands.

Additional resources

Cancerbacup produce an excellent leaflet for patients and partners called *Sexuality and Cancer*. The section entitled 'Some solutions to sexual problems caused by cancer and its treatment' addresses mismatch in desire, pain during intercourse, vaginal dryness and pain, erectile problems and body image problems. You will learn a lot of helpful practical solutions from reading the publication. Read it and be prepared to answer questions. Don't just give it to the patient! It can be downloaded from: http://www.cancerbacup.org.uk/info/sex/sex-5.htm

The least you need to know

⌘ Broach the subject with patients.
⌘ Listen attentively to the patient's story.
⌘ Explore feelings and their relationship to issues such as loss and coping.
⌘ Offer simple advice.
⌘ Refer for additional advice and support if necessary.

References

Annon J (1976) *The Behavioural Treatment of Sexual Problems: Brief therapy*. Harper and Row, New York

Fossa SD, Woehre H, Kurth KH (1997) Influence of urological morbidity on quality of life in patients with prostate cancer. *European Urology* **31** (supplement 3): 3–8

Gamlin RD (1999) Sexuality: a challenge for nursing practice. *Nurs Times* **95**(7): 48–51

Gamlin RD, Sutherland N (1999) Sexuality and advanced illness. In: Lugton J, Kindlen M, eds. *Palliative Care: The Nursing Role*. Churchill Livingstone, Edinburgh

Juraskova I, Butow P, Robertson R, Sharpe L, McLeod C, Hacker N (2003) Post-treatment sexual readjustment following cervical and endometrial cancer: A qualitative insight. *Psycho-oncology* **12**: 267–79

Roper N, Logan W, Tierney A (1980) *The Elements of Nursing*. Churchill Livingstone, Edinburgh

Savage J, ed (1987) *Nurses, Gender and Sexuality*. Heinemann, London

Wells P (2002) No sex please, I'm dying. A common myth explored. *Eur J Palliative Care* **9**(3): 119–22

Chapter links to the NMC's *Code of Professional Conduct* (2002)

2. Respect the patient or client as an individual
    2.1 Partnership in care
    2.2 Promote and respect dignity
    2.4 Help patient's gain access to information and support

3. Obtain consent before you give any treatment or care
    3.1 The right to information
    3.2 Respect for autonomy

5. Protect confidential information
    5.1 Respect the use of information and guard against breaches of confidentiality
    5.2 Seek patient's wishes to share information

Chapter 12

Care priorities in the last days of life

Sister asked me to sit with this elderly man who was unconscious and dying, because he had no known family. I was nineteen on my first ward as a student and full of macho confidence, but this scared the hell out of me. I sat behind the curtain reading the newspaper wondering what to do next. Eventually, I turned to face him and watched his flickering eyes and his changing expressions. I reached over the bed, held his hand and moments later he squeezed my hand hard. I nearly wet myself, but stayed by his side. He died peacefully about ten minutes later still holding my hand.

One of the most significant issues in acute sector care in the UK, where up to 60% of people die is the difficulty staff have in changing the focus of care away from curative medical interventions to a more palliative approach (Clark *et al*, 1997). Within this scenario it can be equally as difficult to moderate that focus once again towards the more terminal phase of life. Those last few days and hours, require a subtle, but significant change in the approach to care, wherever that care takes place. This chapter shows how to achieve this orientation that is so crucial to the quality of the short life that is left to those being cared for. Not all the good practice offered is suitable to all environments, but we are sure that you will find a wide range of options that are achievable within most settings.

The aims of the nursing management

1. The relief of distressing symptoms fears and anxieties in dying patients as far as possible.
2. The provision of active support and encouragement for informal caregivers of dying patients.
3. Enabling patients to die in the place of their choosing, wherever possible, and with a sense of dignity, as they perceive it.
4. Minimising the potential for a complex grief reaction associated with bereavement.

The guiding principles in the terminal phase of care

⌘ Patient and family participation where possible.
⌘ A collaborative multidisciplinary approach by all relevant health professionals.
⌘ Use of appropriate medications, tailored to each person, given regularly to relieve and prevent symptoms.
⌘ Continued regular review of all care over the twenty-four-hour period.
⌘ Access and early referral to specialist services for patient and family support if needed.
⌘ Support and acknowledge the uncertainty of how and when someone may actually die.

Assessment of patient needs

This should involve:

⌘ Enquiry of the patient's perceived symptoms. A holistic approach should be followed.
⌘ Remember the level of detail should be dictated by the patient's condition.
⌘ Remember that patients frequently under-report problems.

The most commonly reported physical symptoms are:

- pain
- dyspnoea
- nausea/vomiting
- agitation/restlessness
- confusion
- noisy breathing
- urinary incontinence or retention
- dry or sore mouth.

It is the professional duty of the nurse to develop a good rapport with the patient and relatives so that such symptoms can be recognised quickly and dealt with accordingly. Whilst prescription of proprietary medication is the responsibility of the doctor, the bulk of care delivered thereafter is a nursing responsibility.

Nursing duties

Physical

- ⌘ Examination of any sites of pain, including duration and intensity of pain by use of a recognised pain assessment tool.
- ⌘ Monitor pressure areas and any aids currently in use. Pressure relieving mattresses will help minimise the risk of skin breakdown, but do not take away the need for careful repositioning. The patient needs to be kept clean and dry.
- ⌘ Careful positioning will help avoid pressure sores and minimise pain from stiff, uncomfortable joints.
- ⌘ Check the mouth regularly for cleanliness and signs of infection. Clean the mouth with a toothbrush whenever possible and offer crushed ice if appropriate. If lips are dry apply a thin coat of Vaseline. Use pineapple chunks to moisten the mouth. These will also assist in cleansing the mouth due to the enzymes within the pineapple juice
- ⌘ The skin: washing the patient and applying moisturising lotion will avoid dry skin. Gentle massage of the hands or feet using either moisturising lotion or diluted aromatherapy oils will aid relaxation and give comfort.

Psychological

Perhaps one of the most poorly addressed and undervalued areas of nursing assessment, yet for the patient often the one most closely associated with their suffering (Becker, 2001).

- ⌘ A patient may fear that the pain they are experiencing could escalate into extreme agony. Some patients resist falling asleep for fear of stopping breathing in their sleep.
- ⌘ The increasing dependency of the dying person which might overwhelm the family, depending on the support available wherever the patient is being cared for.
- ⌘ Past experiences, especially of relatives or friends, who may not have had a peaceful or dignified death.
- ⌘ Preferences about treatment and a feeling of loss of control.
- ⌘ Concerns about treatment, such as morphine accelerating death.

Spiritual

⌘ Awareness of a person's cultural perceptions and belief systems about death and dying is important.

⌘ Anxiety regarding the diagnosis if unknown. Remember that this may be the patient's choice.

⌘ Profound questions asked about death and meaning in life. This is normal and to be expected, as it represents a search for meaning to the event unfolding before them

⌘ Is there overwhelming, uncontrollable distress which is usually associated with severe weakness. It is the fear of losing control that is central to most anxiety in those dying.

⌘ There may be unresolved conflict, or guilt between the family and the dying person.

⌘ Fears about how they will die and what happens after.

Good practice at the bedside

The consciousness level

Most people who die an expected death slip in and out of consciousness over several days, therefore:

⌘ Speak to the patient slowly and clearly, informing them of procedures before carrying them out.

⌘ Speak to the relatives where appropriate and warn them of fluctuating consciousness and the possibility of disorientation and restlessness. Reassure them that it is a normal part of the dying process and is not indicative of poor symptom control.

⌘ Resist full body washes unless absolutely necessary in those hours immediately before death. Such washes are inappropriate in most cases.

⌘ Be sure to keep the bedclothes loose.

⌘ Stop oral fluids when consciousness fluctuates and be sure to say why this is important to the relatives, ie. to prevent fluids being given inappropriately.

⌘ Have sips of water plus ice cubes available and maintain good mouth care.

⌘ Intravenous and subcutaneous infusions should be taken down unless for a clear purpose, ie. hyperkalcaemia. This is a sensitive issue and medical staff should be challenged to justify the rationale behind maintaining IV or subcutaneous fluids close to death. There is an increasing body of evidence that such invasive procedures can exacerbate dyspnoea and are of no benefit to the patient (Ellershaw *et al* 1995; Dunphy *et al*, 1995; Gray, 1999). Do not fall into the trap of condoning such practise merely because it appeases the relatives or medical staff.

Respiration

⌘ Turn the patient from side to side at regular intervals to facilitate the drainage of secretions, but remember it is not advisable to move the patient when death is imminent.

⌘ Leaving the patient on their back may cause the tongue to sag and result in a distressing snoring sound.

⌘ Keep the nose and mouth scrupulously clean.

⌘ Reassure the relatives that the shallow breathing they may be witnessing is not the person gasping for air but a normal aspect of dying.

⌘ Sometimes the relatives may observe long pauses between breathes of up to thirty seconds (Cheyne Stokes Breathing). If this begins to occur reassure the relatives that this is a normal aspect of the dying process to alleviate their anxiety. Because of the intermittent nature of the breaths it can make determining the exact time of death quite difficult, therefore it is good practice that the nursing staff are close by during this period.

Cardiovascular system

⌘ Monitor the patient's pulse discreetly and regularly. When death is imminent the pulse changes to become weaker and more rapid as the heart attempts to compensate for lack of oxygen.

⌘ Encourage the relatives to check the patient's wrist pulse. This is easily done and can provide an early warning to the family of the impending death. If there are family nearby having a break then they can be contacted.

⌘ Change the bed linen and clothing as necessary.

⌘ Tepid sponging can help to cool the patient who is sweating. This is a normal physiological reaction as the body attempts to cool itself to compensate for the slow shutting down of the lungs and the kidneys.

⌘ Light clothing and fresh air circulating is helpful.

⌘ Do not put on extra blankets because the patient feels cold to the touch as this can cause restlessness.

The senses

- ⌘ Try to maximise natural light wherever possible and to avoid the overuse of fluorescent strip lights even though this may be difficult in a hospital situation.
- ⌘ Keep the lights on in the patient's room. Visual acuity deteriorates as a normal part of dying and the patient may wish to be physically close to their family.
- ⌘ Advise visitors to sit next to the patient and not at the end of the bed.
- ⌘ Remove obtrusive furniture and equipment where possible to allow the family uncluttered access to the patient.
- ⌘ Encourage conversation to be in normal tones and not whispers as the sense of hearing can remain acute right up to death.
- ⌘ Artificial tears can help to prevent corneas drying.
- ⌘ Keep all dressings clean and secure.
- ⌘ Use aromatherapy oils to promote a relaxing atmosphere and to help mask bad odours.
- ⌘ Do not use spray deodorisers around the bedside as they can cause coughing and restlessness.

Caring for the relatives

As death approaches:

- ⌘ Encourage them to touch, hold and talk to their loved one.
- ⌘ Explain that hearing is the last sense to be lost even if the person appears unresponsive.
- ⌘ If several relatives are there, encourage some to take a break away from the bedside, but to remain close by and contactable.
- ⌘ Be sure to keep them supplied with drinks and snacks if you can.
- ⌘ Encourage them to do small things for their loved one, eg. combing hair, cleaning the face.
- ⌘ Explain the signs of impending death to the family, where appropriate, with sensitivity. Remember that not all families require or request this; it is a matter of careful judgement on the nurse's part whether this is the correct course of action.
- ⌘ Reassure them that the death itself will be peaceful.

At the moment of death and soon afterwards:

⌘ Provide the family with time, space and privacy to stay with the deceased for as long as they wish.

⌘ Encourage them to touch and hold the deceased reassuring them that the body does not deteriorate quickly.

⌘ Encourage them to say goodbye and to express their feelings if they can. Open grief at this moment is both healthy and appropriate, but people often need permission from the professionals to express themselves.

⌘ Remain discreetly in the background, but available if needed.

⌘ Remember they may be bewildered about what to do next, therefore be sure to have the correct local procedure at hand, backed up with literature if possible.

⌘ Don't forget that the eyes may not close at death so be prepared. Do not use any form of tape or coins to close the eyes as this may damage the tissues. Damp cotton wool balls are the simplest and most effective solution.

Professional duties after a death

⌘ Make sure that the key staff involved know what is happening.

⌘ If organ donation is an issue, know how to contact the team concerned.

⌘ If death is within twenty-four hours of surgery, anaesthetic, or any invasive procedure the coroner needs to be informed. Do not remove cannulae, tubes, or pack orifices before talking to the doctor concerned. If in doubt seek advice from a senior nurse.

⌘ If body donation is arranged know where the university medical school concerned can be contacted.

⌘ If a different culture is concerned know where you can contact the appropriate community leader or minister. Do not assume that the family want this. Establish what rituals need to be observed before and after death with the body and who can be involved.

⌘ Be clear about last offices procedure. This will not be discussed in this chapter as local procedures vary greatly around the country. Please refer to your local policy.

⌘ Remember that as a junior staff member you may not have been involved in this before, so recognise your vulnerability here and seek support.

⌘ Recognise the team's emotional needs at this time also. Help arrange support.

Hospital specific issues in terminal care

⌘ Prescription of adequate doses of analgesia and other medications on a regular basis. Junior medical staff in particular need support and guidance.

⌘ Appropriate information for patients and relatives.

⌘ Recognition of the impact of death on the other patients in a ward. If a patient has been in a four- or six-bed bay for some time, they will almost certainly have formed relationships with those around them. It is both courteous and sensitive to the memory of the deceased to acknowledge the event to these people at an appropriate time.

⌘ Careful handling of requests for postmortem and transplantation.

⌘ Support for relatives when they return to pick up patient's belongings after the death.

⌘ Multi-professional decision when dealing with the transition to terminal care.

⌘ Careful decision-making regarding patient transfer to a hospice or specialist unit.

⌘ Support for junior medical staff who often bear the brunt of breaking bad news as well as patient and family requests for information.

⌘ Support in the clinical area for nursing staff who may have formed a continuing relationship with both patient and relatives.

Home-related issues in terminal care

Inform families and sometimes patients about the signs of the terminal phase, for example:

- increasing tiredness/sleeping
- confusion and/or restlessness
- decreased intake of food and fluids
- incontinence
- diminished urine output
- 'rattling' breathing
- skin mottling.

NB: Avoid telling patients and families that death is like 'falling asleep'.

Inform families about the signs of imminent death, for example:

- patient cannot be roused by shaking or shouting

- patient stops breathing
- death is usually peaceful, not loud or violent
- profound skin pallor develops within half an hour of death.

Instruct families about what to do when the patient dies, for example:

- do not attempt to resuscitate or dial for an emergency ambulance. (ambulance crews are obliged to begin resuscitation and take the body to the nearest hospital — this will be distressing for the family)
- phone for the GP or appropriate local GP on call service
- stress that there is no urgency about contacting an undertaker
- encourage the family to spend time with the body and to actively say goodbye
- inform the family about what reactions to expect and how to cope with extremes of emotional outburst or the reactions of children.

References

Becker R (2001) How will I cope: Psychological aspects of advanced illness. In: Gamlin R, Kinghorn S, eds. *Palliative Nursing: Bringing comfort and hope*. Ballière Tindall, Edinburgh

Clark D, Hockley J, Ahmedzai S, eds (1997) *New Themes in Palliative Care*. Oxford University Press, Oxford

Ellershaw J, Sutcliffe J, Saunders C (1995) Dehydration and the dying patient. *J Pain Symptom Management* **10**(3): 192–7

Dunphy K *et al* (1995) Rehydration in palliative care: if not — why not? *Palliative Med* **9**: 221–8

Gray R (1999) To hydrate or not to hydrate? *Nurs Times* **95**(23): 36–7

National Council for Hospices and Specialist Palliative Care Services (1997) *Changing Gear: Guidelines for Managing the Last Days of Life*. Clinical Guidelines Working Party, December 1997

Useful websites

National Council for Hospice and Specialist Palliative Care Services
http://www.hospice-spc-council.org.uk/

The Scottish Partnership Agency for Palliative and Cancer Care
http://www.spapcc.demon.co.uk/

Chapter links to the NMC's *Code of Professional Conduct* (2002)

2. Respect the patient or client as an individual
   2.1 Partnership in care
   2.2 Promote and respect dignity
   2.4 Help patient's gain access to information and support

3. Obtain consent before you give any treatment or care
   3.1 The right to information
   3.2 Respect for autonomy
   3.6 Competency and advance statements
   3.11 The safe use of complimentary therapies

4. Cooperate with others in the team
   4.3 Communicate your skill, knowledge and expertise
   4.4 Ensure accurate record keeping

5. Protect confidential information
   5.1 Respect the use of information and guard against breaches of confidentiality
   5.2 Seek patient's wishes to share information

6. Maintain your professional knowledge and competence
   6.5 Deliver care based on evidence, research and best practice